HEALTH EDUCATION PLANNING
A Diagnostic Approach

HEALTH EDUCATION PLANNING

A Diagnostic Approach

LAWRENCE W. GREEN

MARSHALL W. KREUTER

SIGRID G. DEEDS

KAY B. PARTRIDGE

with the assistance of
EDWARD BARTLETT

THE JOHNS HOPKINS UNIVERSITY

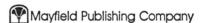Mayfield Publishing Company

**To Bill Griffiths and others
who laid the foundation upon which we built**

Copyright © 1980 by Mayfield Publishing Company
First edition 1980

Library of Congress Catalog Card Number: 79-89920
International Standard Book Number: 0-87484-471-1

Manufactured in the United States of America
Mayfield Publishing Company, 285 Hamilton Avenue, Palo Alto, California 94301

This book was set in Bembo and Avant Garde Book by the Lienett Company and was
printed and bound by R. R. Donnelley and Sons. Sponsoring editor was C. Lansing Hays,
Carole Norton supervised editing, and Judy Chaffin was manuscript editor. Michelle
Hogan supervised production, and the book was designed by Nancy Sears, with cover
design by Bill Nagel. The authors' preparation of this book was supported in part by NIH
grant No.1-T-32-HL0710-02.

Contents

Preface

THIS BOOK IS THE PRODUCT of a period of growth and development in health education that was at times exhilarating but often painful in the recognition that the field has been without a clear articulation of its boundaries, its methods, and its procedures. Only the philosophy and the intellectual roots of health education were sufficiently understood to appear in textbook form. Over several decades, of course, many articles have been published in which practical implications for health education have been derived from specific philosophies, theories, experiences, and occasionally, studies. Only a few of these derived practices have survived long-term analysis and evaluation. From a sociological perspective health education has been more a movement or a series of successive movements than a single profession. Transforming health education principles from philosophical terms to operational ones has been difficult at times. Health education knowledge has been inadequately codified. And the training of health educators has been relatively devoid of uniformity or consistent standards. Outstanding programs have been emulated but often without a supporting understanding of their backgrounds, their methods, or their results.

Practitioners in various professions have struggled, often without clear guidelines, to systematize their planning, delivery, and evaluation of health or educational programs. To avoid the philosophical trap that has caught such previous efforts to codify the practice of health education, we have in this book sought strenuously to minimize the entrapment of method in philosophy. The methods we propose are not entirely value free, and certainly they reflect the main traditions of health education practice; but we have tried to present the methodology in such a way as to be acceptable to people who approach the practice of health education from various philosophical vantage points. It is unavoidable, of course, that our philosophy would inform the presentation throughout, so we might as well state our single overriding principle at the outset. The overriding principle in our approach to health education is that health behavior must be voluntary behavior. Health behavior should be compelled only in those cases when the health of others is threatened. Health means different things to different people, serves different purposes for different people, and is more or less important to different people. Because of this, it is impossible to justify the imposition of rigid criteria of appropriate health behavior unless a behavior has been judged by society as a whole to be a sufficient hazard to the common good to warrant the curtailment of individual choice.

The idea of voluntary behavior has a number of corollaries. First, for example, the reason for a behavior change must be understood by those whose behavior is in question. To accommodate this necessity, we have built into our model of health education a process to ensure agreement between health practitioners and health education recipients (whether individual or group) on the definition of health-related problems. Second, a recommended behavior must be compatible with the values or value system of the concerned person or community. If it is not, then there must be an opportunity to adjust the value system. These and other corollaries of the definition of health education in terms of voluntary behavior have influenced the form and procedures in the framework for planning we propose.

This framework is called PRECEDE (which stands for "predisposing, reinforcing, and enabling causes in educational diagnosis and evaluation") to draw attention to the necessity of asking what behavior precedes each health benefit and what causes precede each health behavior that must be addressed in a health education plan. We have built the framework out of the variety of projects in which it has been developed or tested. We have adjusted it in our teaching and consultation as it has been applied to an ever-widening range of problems in the health field. And, as this goes to press, refinements are still being worked. Even so, we can say with confidence that overall the framework and the procedures that substantiate it are serviceable in a variety of populations with a variety of problems. Hundreds of professionals who have tried it in in-service training programs and subsequently in their work, have attested to the utility of the framework. Additional hundreds of graduate and postgraduate students, including those in the fields of nursing, medicine, health education, pharmacy, dietetics, and dentistry, have demonstrated their ability to understand the framework and apply the procedures in the preparation of project proposals, some of which were taken into the field and subsequently implemented, some of which were funded by government agencies and foundations, and some of which are published as Appendix B of this book.

ACKNOWLEDGMENTS

We are indebted to many people and institutions besides the students and professionals alluded to above. To some we owe an intellectual debt that we have acknowledged in earlier publications of the framework but should mention again here, because we have not attempted to document in this book the source of each of our ideas. The general layout of the framework was inspired first by the work of Ronald Anderson on the utilization of health services and of J. Mayone Stycos on couples' adoption of family planning methods. Not so easily identified is the contribution of our teachers at Berkeley, where the social-psychological approach to health education of Dorothy Nyswander and William Griffith and the sociological orientation of Beryl Robert influenced our approach to problem solving. Our colleagues and graduate students at Johns Hopkins have refined the framework and, in some instances, have published their own elaborations of it with applications to specific situations. These include Anne Ackerman, Peggy Brooks-Bertram, Judith Chwalow, Sharon Dorfman, Lawrence Egbert, Thomas Elwood, Ruth Faden, Donald Fedder, Robert Feldman, Andrew Fisher, Pearl German, Barbara Hebert, Howard Kalmer, David Levine, Carol Lewis, Frances Lewis, Lois Maimon, Joyce Mamon, Barbara Rimer, Debra Roter, Edgar Roulhac, Juliette Sayegh, Melvyn Thorne, Virginia Wang, William Ward, Richard Windsor, Joan Wolle, and Tsering Yangdon.

Many helpful comments have been received on drafts of this manuscript from these and other colleagues, postdoctoral fellows, students, and people who attended our courses and summer workshops. Particularly helpful have been Joshua Adeniyi, Cathy Becker, Robert Bertera, Elisa Braver, Lawren D'Altroy, Monique Julien-Dube, Beth Ewy, Alan Fertziger, Joan

Fink, Brian Flynn, Stuart Fors, Andrea Gielen, Josephine Gimble, Janice Gordon, Walter Gunn, Ann Harvey, Alan Henderson, Caroline Hochreiter, Michael Hosokawa, Elizabeth Howze, Ebenezer Israel, Barbara Jackman, Beverly Jones, William Jones, Jr., JoAnn Kairys, Peter LeBrun, Laurie Liskin, Peggy McManus, Teri Manes, Shelley Meriweather, Jacqueline Miller, Donald Morisky, Patricia Mullen, Fran Owen, Arlene Perino, Marge Petty, Petra Reyes, Anne Rogal, Zora Salisbury, Vicki Sanders, Wendy Squyres, Susan Talty, Mary Taylor, Kathy Tierman, Jeanne Upshaw, Joanne Wayne, Robert Willis, Nan Wolf, and Jane Zapka.

We are particularly grateful for the encouragement of Lansing Hays and the careful, intelligent editing of Judith Chaffin provided by Mayfield Publishing Company. Without his encouragement, this book would not have been written, and without her editing it would not have been read.

Health Education Planning: Key Terms

attitude A relatively constant feeling, predisposition, or set of beliefs directed toward an object, person, or situation.

behavior An action that has a specific frequency, duration, and purpose, whether conscious or unconscious.

behavioral diagnosis Delineation of the specific health actions that can most likely effect a health outcome.

behavioral objective A statement of desired outcome that indicates who is to demonstrate how much of what behavior by when.

belief A statement or sense, declared or implied, intellectually and/or emotionally accepted as true by a person or group.

benefits Valued health outcomes or improvements in quality of life that there is reasonable evidence to believe are causally related to health-care processes.

community   Any collective of people sharing a set of common values.

compliance   Adherence to a prescribed therapeutic or preventive regimen.

culture   The sum of values transmitted over time in a community.

diagnosis   Health or behavioral information that designates the "problem" and its status and information needed for planning and evaluating programs or establishing a prognosis. A *health problem* can be a symptom or complaint, an abnormal physical or laboratory finding, a confirmed diagnosis, or a potential or real threat to physical or emotional well-being.

educational diagnosis   The delineation of factors that predispose, enable, and reinforce a specific health behavior.

educational tool   Any material (such as a bulletin board, leaflet, or videotape) designed to aid learning and teaching through sight and sound; used interchangeably with *educational aids, educational materials,* and *audiovisual aids.*

effectiveness   The extent to which benefits that could be achieved under optimal conditions are achieved in practice.

efficacy   The extent to which an intervention can be shown to be beneficial under optimal conditions.

efficiency   The proportion of total costs (e.g., money, resources, time) that can be related to benefits achieved in practice.

enabling factor   Any characteristic of the environment that facilitates health behavior and any skill or resource required to attain the behavior. (Absence of the characteristic or skill blocks the health behavior.)

epidemiological diagnosis   The delineation of the extent, distribution, and causes of a health problem in a defined population.

evaluation   The process of determining the value or degree of success in achieving a predetermined objective. It usually includes at least the following steps: formulation of the objective, identification of the criteria to be used in measuring success, and determination and explanation of the degree of success. Evaluation is defined more broadly as the comparison of an object of interest against a standard of acceptability.

Health Belief Model   A paradigm used to predict and explain health behavior based on value-expectancy theory.

health education   Any designed combination of methods to facilitate voluntary adaptations of behavior conducive to health.

health outcomes   Any medically or epidemiologically defined characteristic of a patient or health problem in a population that results from health promotion or care provided or required as measured at one point in time.

interventions   The part of a strategy, incorporating method and technique, that actually interacts with a patient or population.

need   (1) Whatever is required for well-being or (2) a requirement an individual or group becomes aware of when values are acquired that demand certain levels of comfort or wellness.

objective   A defined result of specific health activity to be achieved in a finite period of time. Objectives are stated as definite aims or goals of action; they are quantitatively measurable; achievement is reflected in standards of performance. Objectives state (1) who, (2) will experience what change or benefit, (3) how much, and (4) how soon.

planning   The process of establishing priorities, diagnosing causes of problems, and allocating resources to achieve objectives.

predisposing factor   Any characteristic of a patient, consumer, or community that motivates behavior related to health.

priority   Alternatives ranked according to effectiveness or value (importance) or both.

program   A set of planned activities over time designed to achieve specified objectives.

program effectiveness   The extent to which preestablished program objectives are attained as a result of program activity.

program efficiency   The proportion of resources used in the actual attainment of objectives relative to the total resources expended.

program objective   A statement of desired outcome that indicates who is to obtain how much of what benefits at what point in time following the implementation of a plan.

quality assessment   Measurement of practice for comparison with accepted standards to determine the degree of excellence.

quality assurance   Formal process of implementing quality assessment and quality improvement.

quality of life   The perception of individuals or groups that their needs are being satisfied and that they are not being denied opportunities to achieve happiness and fulfillment.

reinforcing factor   Any reward or punishment following or anticipated as a consequence of a health behavior.

screening   A technology designed to select from a large number of people those individuals with signs or symptoms requiring further diagnosis and, if indicated, treatment.

social diagnosis   The assessment in both objective and subjective terms of high-priority problems, defined for a population in terms of economics, work, unemployment, illegitimacy, civic disturbance, and the like, and for an individual in terms of quality of life.

social indicator   A quality the change in the numerical value of which is expected, all other things being equal, to reflect a change in the quality of life.

social problem   A situation that a significant number of people believe to be a source of difficulty or unhappiness. A social problem consists of an objective situation as well as a social interpretation.

strategy   A plan of action that anticipates barriers and resources in relation to achieving a specific objective.

tactic   A method or approach employed as a part of a strategy.

value   A preference shared and transmitted within a community.

1

Health Education Today and the PRECEDE Framework

THESE ARE REWARDING TIMES for health professionals who have been committed to the concept of health education. A sudden emergence of public and professional interest in health education is being fueled by national and international trends converging on the issues of self-help, prevention, and health promotion. Recent legislative and related activity suggests that the interest is more than sentiment and rhetoric. The Health Maintenance Organization Act, which became law in 1973, specified that preventive and educational services were mandatory for health maintenance organizations receiving federal certification.[1] In 1973, the President's Committee on Health Education advocated the establishment of a Bureau of Health Education in the Department of Health, Education and Welfare and, in the private sector, a National Center for Health Education. Both are now active as national focal points for action. The National Health Planning and Resource Development Act of 1974[2] specified public health education as one of the health priorities of the

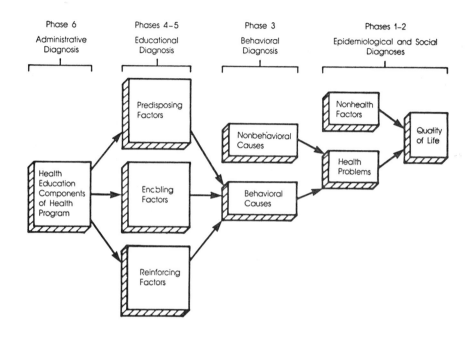

Phase 6	Phases 4–5	Phase 3	Phases 1–2
Administrative Diagnosis	Educational Diagnosis	Behavioral Diagnosis	Epidemiological and Social Diagnoses

nation. In 1976, PL 94-317[3] established an Office of Health Information and Health Promotion under the Assistant Secretary of Health in the Department of Health, Education and Welfare. In the spring of 1978, the Bureau of Health Manpower sponsored a national gathering of health educators for the purpose of establishing criteria for possible use in the certification of health educators.

In addition to these activities, other trends can be noted. The literature indicates that innovative programs are being tested in community, school, patient, and occupational settings; and there is evidence of increased interest and participation in self-care and self-help groups.[4] Canada's "Operation Lifestyle" is an example of the commitment of an entire nation to prevention and health education.[5]

Health Education in Europe, a report published in 1976, provides an overview of health education policies, trends, and practices in twenty-eight countries. In summarizing the report Schnocks states, "everywhere in Europe today, health education is perceived as an integral dimension of health care and an essential prerequisite to effective legislative action aimed at protecting people from health hazards. It is also recognized that modern health policy calls for educational interventions which have a sound scientific foundation."[6]

Several interesting examples of health education innovations are cited in the report, including a comprehensive cardiovascular disease program in North Karelia, Finland, and a twenty-five-year prospective study in Sweden designed to curb smoking by means of selected social influences.

D. N. Loransky, Director of the USSR's Central Institute for Scientific Research in Health Education explains that the Presidium of the Academy of Medical Sciences of the USSR identified health education as a factor of national significance and established a special health education problem commission in 1976, calling it a decision that "heralds a new and important period in the development of health education in the country: from now on, all the medical departments and institutes located in the various republics and regions will participate in educational activities on a regular and planned basis.[7]

Although international funding for health education is still extremely limited, the trend may be changing. Recent support for several large-scale demonstrations and experimental trials suggests a growing interest in research into the effects of health education.[8] At all levels—legislative, administrative, professional, and consumer—there is tangible evidence of a strengthening commitment to health education.

THE GOAL: QUALITY HEALTH EDUCATION

There are almost as many definitions of *health education* as there are health educators. The definition offered by the President's Committee on Health Education is representative: "Health education is a process which bridges the gap between health information and health practices. Health education motivates the person to take the information and do something with it––to keep himself healthier by avoiding actions that are harmful and by forming habits that are beneficial."[9]

This definition suggests, as do virtually all the others, that health education is related to health *behavior* either in helping* people to maintain their

---

*The terms *helping* and *facilitating* are preferable to *motivating,* as used in the definition. Health education cannot motivate behavior in the formal psychological sense. Motivation is not something done *to* people; it is a drive that occurs within the individual. Health education can strengthen and appeal to existing motives and can enable the behavioral expression of existing motives, but it does not "motivate."

life-styles or in helping them to develop their life-styles in health-enhancing directions. Ethical and political issues are raised right away when one begins to consider altering behavior. These must be addressed, and it is best done *before* intervention by means of mutual diagnosis and planning between health educators as change agents and patients, students, workers, or consumers as those contemplating change.

Mutual planning and diagnosis implies *process,* another important aspect of the committee definition. Health education as process means that health education activities have a common basis no matter *where* they occur, whether in clinical, community, school, home, or work settings. Emphasizing process makes it possible to avoid being diverted by dissimilarities of settings and of educational content and methods and to keep goals more clearly in focus. Sliepcevich, in a report to a national workshop studying the certification of health educators in the United States, urged patient, community, and school health educators not to "let territorial imperatives in the titles (school, community, patient) interfere with our common goal of education for health."[10] Our emphasis in this text will be on the common steps that precede intervention in clinical, school, and community health education.

As enthusiasm for health education gains momentum worldwide, and as public and professional interest turn to commitment, one can most certainly expect more intense attention to be paid to questions of performance and accountability, especially when public funds are allocated. While there are many who are counting the potential cost savings of health education, others have been more cautious. Richards, in his comprehensive review of methods and efficacy in health education, warned: "All too often campaigns which were never properly designed or conducted are termed failures but the exact reason for these disappointments never charted. . . . It is well for us to note that in many problem areas there is a lack of a firm methodological basis on which to plan experimental interventions."[11]

Knowles, a recognized advocate of health promotion and preventive medicine who cites the need for quality school health education as a top priority for public policy in prevention, levied the following criticism at school health programs. His view, though exaggerated, is not unusual: "School health programs are abysmal at best, confining themselves to peremptory sick calls and posters on brushing teeth and eating three meals a day; there are no examinations to determine if anything's been learned. Awareness of danger to body and mind is not acquired until the mid-twenties in our culture . . . children tire of 'scrub your teeth,' 'don't eat that junk,' 'leave your dingy alone,' 'go to bed' and 'get some exercise.' "[12]

Systematic program planning and evaluation is essential if health education is to attain validity in the eyes of the public and the health professionals and policy makers who scrutinize its worth.

Unless they have well-defined schemes for health education planning, in which long-range outcomes, behavioral objectives, and program inputs are clearly defined in relation to each other, well-intended health educators run the risk of straying into ritualistic and questionable health education practices. Such practices are called traps. Practitioners fall into the technician trap when they become so involved with "doing" health education that they lose sight of why the program is offered in the first place. Rosenstock saw victims of this trap as losing themselves "in formulating and conducting activities—planning messages of the mass media, using neighborhood organizations to spread messages, designing messages to arouse emotions—all without really thinking out why one is doing these things. And in such cases, it is easy to fall into the trap of substituting activities for objectives."[13]

There is also the technology trap in which health education practice seems to be based on a series of fallacies the sum of which suggests that the answer to effective health education lies entirely in the quality and quantity of advanced educational technology. One of these fallacies is the *empty vessel fallacy*. In this, health educators behave as if all they have to do to ensure the success of their programs is to pour health information into the empty minds of an eagerly awaiting target population.[14] As an extension, technologies are sought that will transmit the most information to the most people by and large regardless of their differing beliefs, attitudes, values, and perceptions.

Another fallacy, creating a different form of technology trap, is the *fallacy of the inherent superiority or inferiority of some methods*. Many practitioners apparently lose sight of the fact that an educational method is only as effective as its *appropriate* application. In such a frame of mind, practitioners are convinced that their methods are the only effective methods for health education. Some work almost exclusively through group process; some believe that television is the only effective means of communication; others believe that mass communication can achieve nothing in behavior change and give their attention to more personal and direct methods. The diagnostic approach to planning health education that we will be presenting recognizes that there is nothing inherently superior or inferior about any method of education. Each has a potential.

The *fallacy of the more, the better* creates a third form of the technology trap. Practitioners sharing this misconception assume that positive outcomes will increase proportionately with more time, more television coverage, more media equipment, more personnel, or more contacts.[15]

As health educators with experience in clinical, community, and school settings, we are sympathetically but painfully aware of the shortcomings of some health education efforts. We are also aware of some very innovative and successful health education efforts, and it is precisely to build on the successes rather than to repeat the failures that we offer in the following chapters the framework and procedures that we call PRECEDE. PRECEDE should be viewed as a tool to use intelligently in drawing on and applying the most appropriate scientific theories and educational technologies in planning effective health education.

THE SCOPE OF HEALTH EDUCATION

We define *health education* as follows: "Health education is any combination of learning experiences designed to facilitate voluntary adaptations of behavior conducive to health."

This definition emphasizes the scope as well as the purpose of health education. It enables us to delineate more sharply than the earlier definition from the President's Committee on Health Education which programs, activities, and methods may be characterized as educational. Most health education activities are not autonomous, free-standing programs in themselves. They are embedded in other programs, and many are not identified as health education. Indeed, a few practitioners sometimes disavow any association with health education in an attempt to distinguish their efforts as more innovative, modern, technological, behavioristic, client-centered, or scientific than they perceive health education to be. Health education programs often are not labeled as such even when the methods employed clearly derive their philosophical, technical, and theoretical or scientific approaches from education, educational psychology, educational technology, or health education itself.

The various labels used for health education programs and activities—motivation programs, behavior modification, health counseling, and communications—illustrate the scope, diversity, and boundaries of educational applications in health.

The term *motivation,* as in *motivation programs,* has been used especially in family planning to refer to the activities generally included in a health education program.[16] Motivation programs are usually combined with "incentive schemes" designed to appeal more directly to economic motives for family limitation.[17] From a formal psychological standpoint, the term *motivation* used in this way is used incorrectly. Motivation is a construct that has reference to the internal dynamics of behavior, not to the external stimuli; hence, motivation programs are correctly identified as programs based on the use of motive-arousing appeals. Motivational strategies qualify as means of health education under our definition as long as motives are not aroused to the point at which behavior is compelled. At that point the condition of voluntary change, essential to our definition, has been violated.

The meaning of the term *behavior modification,* originally used exclusively by behavioral psychologists,[18] has been extended to include a wide range of educational and political strategies for which the primary objectives are changes in behavior.[19] Puristic behavioral psychologists would disallow from application of the term any educational method designed to bring about changes in behavior by means of changes in knowledge or attitudes. But behavior modification techniques qualify as health educational methods as long as the subjects voluntarily submit to them to achieve changes they desire in their own behavior.[20] Some variations of behavior modification methods that are used in educational settings are designed specifically to increase the degree of self-control and self-direction the individual exercises.[21]

The activities associated with the term *health counseling* and its variants (*genetic counseling, diet counseling, patient counseling*) constitute another category of health education insofar as they represent an approach to voluntary change in health behavior. To the degree that emotional disturbance interferes with voluntary control of behavior, counseling is psychotherapeutic rather than educational. Counseling that is more psychotherapeutic than informational in its method and content is outside the scope of health education.

Social psychologists, marketing and public opinion researchers, media specialists, and health educators—all are concerned with mass communications. Communications are used to affect behavior in every sphere of human endeavor.[22] Their use in relation to health behavior is usually within the scope of health education programming,[23] except when they are used to advertise or promote products or causes inconsistent with the health needs of consumers.[24]

The foregoing examples of health education activities not ordinarily labeled as such illustrate the kinds of commonalities and distinctions that need to be attended to in planning programs. We prefer the use of the term *health education* to the narrower and in some instances more insidious alternatives such as *behavior modification* and *patient teaching.* The alternative terms are appropriate to refer to specific techniques or strategies of behavior change but should be associated with health education only when it is clear that the patient or consumer is in voluntary control of the decision to change. Figure 1.1 summarizes the points we have been making, showing the relationship between technologies for behavior change and health education. Note, as we have discussed, the applications of each that do not qualify as means of health education.

The defining characteristic of health education as we see it, then, is the voluntary participation of the consumer in determining his or her own health practices. This is not merely a philosophical tenet. *The evidence that the durability of cognitive and behavioral changes is proportional to the degree of active rather*

FIGURE 1.1

Examples of overlapping technologies for changing health-related behavior

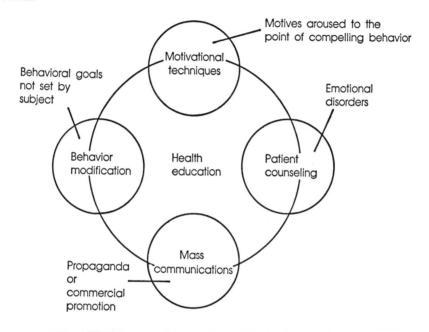

SOURCE: Reprinted with permission from Health Education Monographs, copyright 1978, Society for Public Health Education.

than passive participation of the learner is overwhelming. In addition, there are practical and strategic reasons to emphasize the voluntary nature of health education. It is important to avoid public resistance or reaction to programs that might be perceived as propagandistic, manipulative, coercive, politically or commercially directed, threatening, or paternalistic.

Other forms and methods of health education that define its scope are community organization, in-service training, consultation, group work, computer-assisted instruction, noncomputerized teaching machines and audiovisual methods, patient teaching, health fairs, exhibits, libraries, conferences, and routine health provider-consumer interactions. The scope of health education is defined as much, however, by its expected outcomes as by its methods and forms. And the changes in behavior related to health problems that may come about as a result of health education are numerous and variegated.

FIGURE 1.2

Health education as intervention: Influencing voluntary adoption of
behavior conducive to health

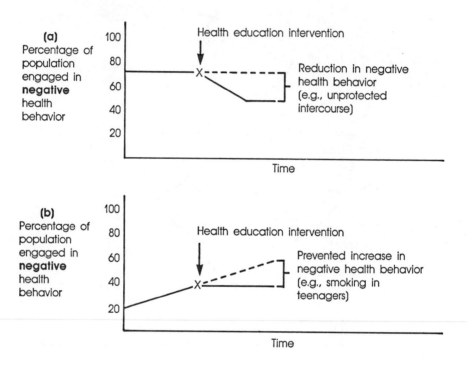

HEALTH EDUCATION AS INTERVENTION:
THE **PRECEDE** FRAMEWORK

Important to the foregoing discussion is the idea of intervention. Organized
health education activity is based on the desire to intervene in the process of
development and change in such a way as to maintain positive health behavior or to interrupt a behavioral pattern that is linked to increased risks for illness, injury, disability, or death. The behavior is usually that of the people
whose health is in question, but often it may be the behavior of those who
control resources or rewards, such as community leaders, parents, employees, peers, teachers, and health professionals as well. Whether a health education program is operating at the primary (hygiene), secondary (early detection), or tertiary (therapeutic) stage of prevention, it may accurately be seen

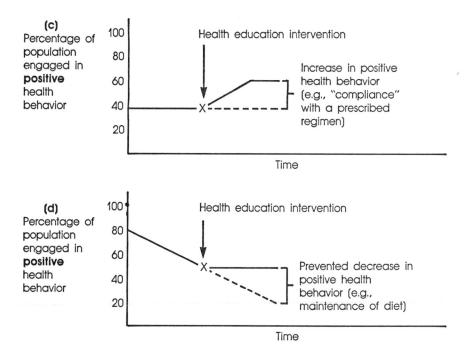

as an intervention, the purpose of which is to short-circuit illness or to enhance the quality of life through change or development of health-related behavior (fig. 1.2). Use of the PRECEDE framework (PRECEDE is an acronym for predisposing, reinforcing, and enabling causes in educational diagnosis and evaluation) will render specific insights concerning evaluation. It will also provide a highly focused target for intervention.

Before going further, we wish to make clear that PRECEDE is not offered as *the* exclusive road to quality health education. It is, however, a theoretically "robust" model that we believe speaks to the acknowledged problem in health education: disjointed planning. It is robust in the sense that it applies to health education in a variety of situations. It has served as a successful model in a number of rigorously evaluated "real world" clinical trials;[25] as a useful guide to the development of local health department programs, adopted by at least two state health departments;[26] as a guide to the review of maternal and

child health projects;[27] as an analytic tool for policy analysis for health education on a national and international scale;[28] and as an organizing framework
for curriculum development in health education for nurses,[29] pharmacists,[30]
and allied health professionals.[31]

Learning to Start from the Other End

Our experience suggests that many people responsible for health education
programs initiate their programs by considering or even designing the actual
intervention to be employed. What's wrong with that? Let us respond by
noting a presumed cause-effect relationship.

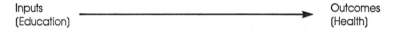

Inputs   Outcomes
(Education)   (Health)

In this schema "inputs" are interventions (or processes), and "outcomes" are the anticipated results of the interventions in terms of changes in
medical or social problems or conditions. Health practitioners, because of
their activist orientation, have an understandable tendency to begin with inputs. After a quick glance at the general problem at hand, they immediately
begin to design and implement the health education intervention and assume
that the outcome will occur automatically.

The PRECEDE framework directs the health educator's initial attention to
outcomes rather than to inputs, forcing him or her to begin the health education planning process from the "outcome" end. It encourages the asking of
why questions before the asking of *how* questions. From the standpoint of
planning, then, what may seem to be the wrong end to start from is, in fact,
the right one. One begins with the final outcome and asks what must precede
that outcome by determing what causes that outcome.

Stated another way, the factors important to an outcome must be diagnosed before the intervention is designed; if they are not, the intervention will
be based on guesswork and runs a greater risk of being misdirected and
ineffective.

The Seven Phases of PRECEDE

Working through PRECEDE is much like solving a mystery. One is led to think
deductively, to start with the final consequences and work back to the original causes. There are seven basic phases in the procedure (fig. 1.3). To provide an overview, they may be superficially described as follows:

Phase 1   Ideally, in the first place, one begins with a consideration of
"quality of life" by assessing some of the general problems of concern to the

people in the population of patients, students, workers, or consumers. The kinds of social problems a given community experiences are good barometers of the quality of life there. What these problems are can be ascertained by several methods that are discussed in some detail in the second chapter.

Phase 2   The task in phase 2 is to identify those specific health problems that appear to be contributing to the social problems noted in phase 1. Using available data and data generated by appropriate investigations together with epidemiological and medical findings, the health educator ranks the several health problems and (using methods suggested in chap. 3) selects the specific health problem most deserving of scarce educational resources.

We should point out here that many health educators, particularly those working in school health education or patient education, will be given the task of developing a program *after* someone else has already gone through phases 1 and 2 and concluded that educational intervention is needed. We appreciate that situation but advise practitioners to be certain that the first two steps have been done well. Such precautionary action ensures that the existing data are valid and also familiarizes the practitioner with crucial foundation information and assumptions.

Phase 3   Phase 3 consists of identifying the specific health-related behaviors that appear to be linked to the health problem chosen as deserving of most attention in phase 2. As these are the behaviors that the intervention will be tailored to affect, it is essential that they be identified very specifically and carefully ranked. Notice in figure 1.3 that we have linked a category called "nonbehavioral factors" to the "health problems" box. Nonbehavioral factors are economic, genetic, and environmental factors. They are acknowledged here because of the power they have, however indirect, to influence health.[32] Being cognizant of such forces will enable educators to be more realistic about the limitations of their programs. It will also enable them to recognize that powerful social forces might be affected when the principles of PRECEDE are applied by well-organized health groups and coalitions on the national level. Even at the local level, health-related behaviors influenced by health education can include collective behavior directed at economic or environmental factors.

Phase 4   On the basis of cumulative research on health behavior,[33] we have identified three "classes" of factors that have potential for affecting health behavior: predisposing factors, enabling factors, and reinforcing factors. Predisposing factors,[34] a person's attitudes, beliefs, values, and perceptions, facilitate or hinder personal motivation for change. Enabling factors may be considered to be barriers created mainly by societal forces or systems. Limited facilities, inadequate personal or community resources, lack of income or health insurance, and even restrictive laws and statutes are examples of enabling factors. The skills and knowledge required for a desired behavior

FIGURE 1.3
The PRECEDE framework

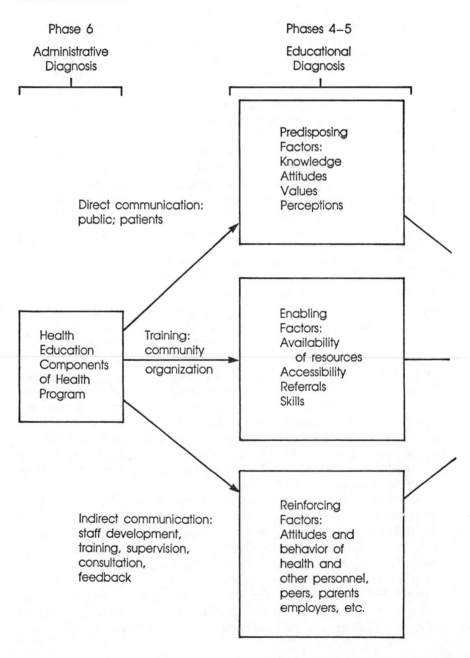

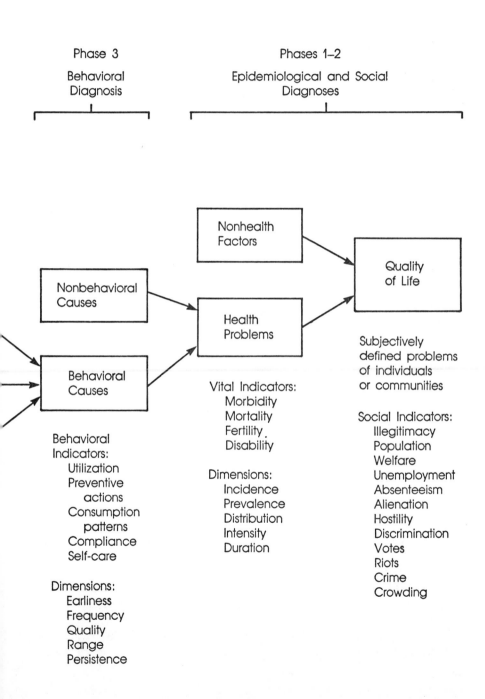

Phase 3

Behavioral
Diagnosis

Phases 1–2

Epidemiological and Social
Diagnoses

Nonhealth
Factors

Quality
of Life

Nonbehavioral
Causes

Health
Problems

Behavioral
Causes

Subjectively
defined problems
of individuals
or communities

Vital Indicators:
  Morbidity
  Mortality
  Fertility.
  Disability

Behavioral
Indicators:
  Utilization
  Preventive
    actions
  Consumption
    patterns
  Compliance
  Self-care

Social Indicators:
  Illegitimacy
  Population
  Welfare
  Unemployment
  Absenteeism
  Alienation
  Hostility
  Discrimination
  Votes
  Riots
  Crime
  Crowding

Dimensions:
  Incidence
  Prevalence
  Distribution
  Intensity
  Duration

Dimensions:
  Earliness
  Frequency
  Quality
  Range
  Persistence

to occur also qualify as enabling factors. Reinforcing factors are those related to the feedback the learner receives from others, the result of which may be either to encourage or to discourage behavioral change.

The fourth phase, then, is sorting and categorizing, according to the three classes just cited, the factors that seem to have direct impact on the behavior selected in phase 2.

Phase 5   Study of the predisposing, enabling, and reinforcing factors automatically takes the educator into the fifth phase of PRECEDE. At this point he or she is called on to decide exactly which of the factors making up the three classes are to be the focus of the intervention. The decision is based on their relative importance and the resources available to influence them.

Phase 6   Armed with pertinent and systematically organized diagnostic information, the health educator is ready for phase 6, which is the actual development and implementation of a program. If he or she keeps firmly in mind the limitations of his or her resources, time constraints, and abilities, the appropriate educational interventions will almost be self-evident from the diagnosis of predisposing, enabling, and reinforcing factors. All that remains is the selection of the right combination of interventions (chap. 6) and an assessment of administrative problems and resources (chap. 7).

Phase 7   Listing evaluation as the last phase is misleading. We consider evaluation to be an integral and continuous part of working with the entire framework. Even though we discuss the evaluation component of PRE-CEDE in considerable detail in chapter 8, criteria for evaluation naturally fall out of the framework during the diagnostic procedure. These are highlighted as we go along. For example, early on in the framework, we will be emphasizing the importance of clearly stating program and behavioral objectives so that the standards of acceptability are defined before rather than after the evaluation.

FOUNDATIONS: STAYING ON SOLID GROUND

The PRECEDE framework for planning is founded on the requirements of four disciplines: epidemiology, social/behavioral sciences, administration, and education. Although one must necessarily draw on all four throughout, each stands as a primary support to a specific phase of PRECEDE. Successful completion of phases 1, 2, and portions of 3 depends heavily on the use of epidemiological methods and information. Working effectively through phases 3 and 4 requires familiarity with social/behavioral theory and concepts. And handling the complex task of designing and implementing a health education program demands knowledge of educational and administrative theory as well as experience. In presenting this framework, we are assuming that the reader has had basic exposure to these several disciplines that constitute the scientific foundation of health education. Throughout work with PRECEDE, two basic propositions are emphasized: (1) health and health behavior are caused by multiple factors; and (2) because health and health behavior are determined by multiple factors, health education efforts to affect behavior must be multidimensional. It is the multidimensional nature of the health education process that demands the kind of professional preparation in which several scientific and professional disciplines are integrated. It is not surprising that educators occasionally become discouraged and even disenchanted as they wade through and try to synthesize biomedical science, behavioral science, and education. The PRECEDE framework can give direction and focus to such attempts at synthesis. The challenge—to pull together a variety of rapidly developing disciplines as a basis for understanding and in some way contributing to improvements in the quality of life—is what sustains commitment to and hope for health education.

EXERCISES

1. What trends have you noticed in recent years in your community or among your friends in health behavior and health concerns? Can you find objective data to support your observations? If not, how would you go about verifying your subjective view of these trends?

2. Identify five or six national or international health campaigns or programs spanning a number of years. How do you account for the public concern with these different health problems at different times? What were the major features of the health education component of these programs? Why have different programs or problems at different times required different health education methods?

3. Identify and describe the demographic characteristics (geographic location, size, age and sex distribution, etc.) of a population (students, patients, workers, residents) whose quality of life you would like to improve. You will follow the population you choose through most of the remaining exercises in this book. Look ahead at these exercises to be sure the population is appropriate for the diagnostic and planning steps required.

2

Social Diagnosis: Assessing Quality of Life Concerns

HEALTH IS NOT in itself an ultimate value; it is, rather, an "instrumental" value. People cherish health because it serves other ends. That the word *health* evades sharp, universally accepted definition is perhaps the best indication we have of its subjective nature. Disease, disability, and discomfort are conditions of life that inform a variety of personal, economic, and social concerns. When there are social problems, we may discover health problems that contribute to them. And underneath every concern alleged to be a health concern is a deeper concern with the things that are threatened by its loss. Awareness of the instrumental nature of health raises a primary question in health education planning: On what basis, and by what process, are decisions made to determine which health problem(s) deserve the highest priority for the investment of limited health education resources?

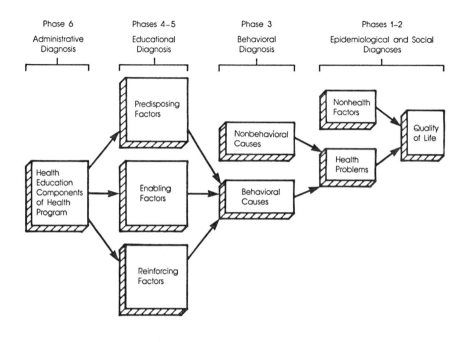

Phase 6	Phases 4–5	Phase 3	Phases 1–2
Administrative Diagnosis	Educational Diagnosis	Behavioral Diagnosis	Epidemiological and Social Diagnoses

ATTENDING TO QUALITY OF LIFE CONCERNS FIRST

The PRECEDE framework is designed so that health education activities are developed and delivered only after the specific, long-range benefits of such activities have been determined. Integral to the sequence is that educators take the time to consider carefully social outcomes or quality of life concerns before plunging into the intricacies of methodology and even before accepting without question the priority assigned to a health problem. Why is this advantageous? There are four reasons.

Increasing Efficiency and Conserving Resources

Focusing on desired outcomes enhances specificity and perspective in planning. Trying to conduct a program with a vague or moving target wastes effort and resources. Working with poorly defined goals creates a "shot in the dark" mentality that leads to diffuse interventions in which scarce educational resources are spread too thinly to have much impact. The chances for appropriate, valid interventions are directly dependent on the clarity and specificity with which the outcomes are defined. Health professionals can undertake program planning more confidently and systematically if they know ultimate program goals in advance.

Informing the "Consumer"

When the objectives are clearly defined and the expected benefits are identified, participants in a program can be given an accurate picture of the stakes before they are asked to change their beliefs or practices. The question of mutual understanding of goals between educator and learner is a practical one, but, beyond that, the ethical issues of informed consent in any behavioral intervention must be considered by all health professionals. Patients and consumers should have the opportunity to weigh the expected benefits of the recommended behavior against the risks and benefits of alternative courses of action.[1]

Evaluating the Results

Initial identification of intended benefits strengthens evaluation. The assessment of benefits is likely to be more efficient and the results more convincing when the desired outcomes are decided before data are collected and the results computed rather than after. Health education is less likely than surgery to get away with the kind of thinking reflected by the half-jocular observation, "The operation was a success but the patient died."[2]

Enhancing a Sense of Purpose

Early focus on outcomes helps health education planners to nurture a broader perspective than that possible if they are just "doing" health education. They are constantly reminded of the reasons that health education is being offered, which gives purpose and meaning to professional practice. The benefits of health education may include improvements not only in health but in other areas of social concern and quality of life as well. When health services must compete with other social services for public support and resources, this perspective is more than philosophically comforting; it is politically sane.[3]

   In the first phase of the PRECEDE process, the planner's task is to understand the social "problems" as patients, consumers, or the community perceive them, to objectify these perceptions, and to establish links between the social problems and the specific health problems that should become the more immediate focus of the health education program. After working through this phase, the planner should be able to state how the alleviation of a given health problem will affect the subjective or social problems that reflect the quality of life of the target population.

HEALTH AND SOCIAL PROBLEMS:
AN INTERACTING RELATIONSHIP

The PRECEDE process is outlined as a one-way cause and effect model. Inputs (health education) will cause certain changes, which will cause other changes, which eventually will lead to outcomes (improved quality of life). The relationships between health and quality of life are not one way only, of course. Figure 2.1 diagrams the relationships between them at the individual and community levels. The arrows suggest that health problems have an impact on quality of life at the same time that quality of life affects health. The top arrow is meant to suggest that social problems influencing the quality of life can lead to health problems, an aspect of the relationship that would be of interest to social workers, recreation professionals, and those shaping health and social policy.[4] The bottom arrow indicates that health problems have an impact on quality of life which interventions for health improvement or maintenance can modify. This is the aspect of the exchange emphasized in PRECEDE; indeed, it is the aspect with which health education practice is primarily concerned. Health education policy is concerned ultimately with the top arrow.

A review of the literature reveals that the concept of quality of life is as difficult to define and measure as the concepts of health and love,[5] even though the reality of all three is widely accepted. In fact, some people question whether it is possible or even advisable to quantify quality of life. They

FIGURE 2.1

The relationship between health and social problems

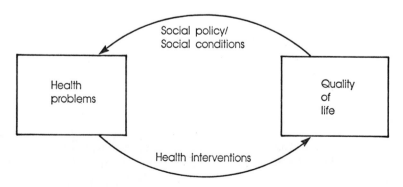

claim that efforts to make explicit and generalize the factors that account for quality of life will necessarily ignore the subtle individual differences in perception within a given population. They also contend that it is inappropriate to impose one person's perception of happiness, satisfaction, and wellness on another who views those same factors differently. While these are important and legitimate issues, it is a fact that the majority of health education programs are delivered in community settings. If we acknowledge the value of community oriented programs, we need to demonstrate their effectiveness in terms of the shared interests of many.[6] As primitive as current quality of life measures are, it is better to initiate the health education planning process with specific understanding of the social condition of the prospective target population than it is to proceed on the basis of informed intuition (what a health professional *thinks* the population needs), national trends, or outright guesswork.

Virtually all attempts to appraise quality of life begin with the study of social problems. An Environmental Protection Agency (EPA) publication, *The Quality of Life Concept: A Potential Tool for Decision-Makers,* defined a *social problem* as "a situation affecting a significant number of people that is believed by them and/or by a significant number of others in the society to be a source of difficulty or unhappiness, and one that is capable of amelioration. Thus, a social problem consists of both an objective situation and a subjective social interpretation."[7] The definition suggests that objective situations and subjective social interpretations will be the two basic components of quality of life indicators. For the purpose of planning, we can extrapolate two ways of generating quality of life indicators. The first consists of identifying the specific factors within a community that can be expressed numerically. Such factors as employment, absenteeism, levels of education, population density, crime rates, discriminatory practices, housing, and social services are examples of factors that can be so expressed.

The second way to determine social indicators is simply to ask members of a target population what they consider to be the major obstacles to improvement in the quality of their lives. Their responses constitute their perceived needs or, in terms of the EPA definition, the subjective social interpretations. Both the objective approach and the subjective approach have been formalized in a variety of methods.[8]

SOME STRATEGIES FOR IDENTIFYING SOCIAL PROBLEMS

Whenever possible, because time and resources are precious, it is economical to retrieve existing information rather than to generate new data. Federal, state, and local offices of housing and urban planning, employment security, law enforcement, and social service agencies all keep reasonably up-to-date records that can serve as excellent sources of relevant information. For a thorough social diagnosis, however, additional data are inevitably needed. They can be gathered in several ways.

Reviewing the Literature

It goes without saying that the biomedical, health education, and behavioral science literature should be the first resource for ideas in health education planning, implementation, and evaluation. By carefully examining the findings and methods of others, the health education planner can gain insights and sharpen his or her ideas of the questions to be asked in a social diagnosis. For example, take the results of a survey done on happiness. A sample population in the Detroit area was asked the simple question: "Taken altogether, how would you say things are these days—would you say you are very happy, pretty happy or not too happy?" The data indicated that the "not too happy" responses were greater among

1. those who lived in Detroit inner city (25 percent) than among those who lived in the suburbs (5 percent)
2. unemployed men (34 percent) than among employed men (8 percent)
3. the poor (15–23 percent) than among the affluent (6–8 percent)[9]

Such data help determine and may help justify the choice of groups or geographic target areas within a specific community to be given first priority for data collection and program planning.

Data from previously done studies may also provide insight into aspects of a social problem that may merit specific attention when the program is implemented. Consider a study of 987 university employees to determine the associations between various dimensions of job satisfaction and health status. Job satisfaction and physical and psychological health were measured by self-reports. Findings were generally consistent with previous studies that examined health status as it relates to a variety of work settings. Health status of college personnel was related to occupational groups: (1) Overall job satisfaction was highest among the highest-status groups (faculty, administration) and lowest among the lowest-status group (secretary, clerk); and (2) the people with the lowest job satisfaction reported more physical health problems and a lower level of psychological well-being.[10]

These studies suggest that questions which generate data regarding general feelings of well-being ("How would you say things are these days?") or more specific aspects of health (the relationship between job satisfaction and health status) can be surprisingly helpful to health educators in the earliest stages of the planning process. Such questions link health problems to social structure, social problems, and social conditions.

The Nominal Group Process

The nominal group process is a method for assessing community perceptions of problems in a way that overcomes many of the traditional problems of unequal representation of opinions. The method consists of a series of small-group procedures designed to compensate for the usual dynamics of social power that emerge in most planning meetings. Those who use the method should keep in mind that its purpose is to identify and rank problems, not to solve them. The method, described as it applies to public health by Van de Ven and Delbecq,[11] is more effective than either the Delphi technique or interaction group process for generating ideas and getting equal participation from group members.[12] Gilmore describes the method as follows:

1. Arrange the participants into groups of six to seven members.

It is important that the size does not exceed seven in order to allow for appropriate interaction. Those selected as participants should be representative of, and knowledgeable about, the community in question.

2. Pose a single question to the group.

It is best if the question can be in writing on a blackboard, flip-chart, or hand-out sheets. As stressed by Delbecq, the question should be generated following consideration for (a) the objective of the meeting, (b) examples of the type of items sought, (c) the development of alternative questions, and (d) the pilot-testing of alternative questions with a sample group. One example of the type of question which has been used by the author is the following: "What do you consider to be the major health problems you are facing at this time?"

3. Have the participants of each small group write down their responses.

Sheets of paper with the question listed at the top can be given out; this provides an easy reference point for the group members. However, if this is not possible, writing the question down on a blackboard, flip-chart, or overhead projector will suffice. Although the actual amount of time necessary to complete this assignment will vary depending upon the particular question which is posed, an approximate amount of time would be 15 minutes. It is important that the group proceed in absolute silence. (This is the responsibility of the group leader.) Such an approach enables the group to reflect carefully upon their ideas, to be motivated by the observance of others who are working diligently by writing down their responses, and to be involved in a competition-free atmosphere where premature decisions do not have to be made.

4. Elicit individual responses in a round-robin fashion.

First, one participant is asked to give a single response, the next gives a single response, and this continues until each participant has contributed a single response. As the responses are stated, they are written by the group leader on a blackboard or flip-chart, each item being given a number (1, 2, 3, etc.). The same process is repeated for a second, then a third time, etc., until all contributions have been recorded. This procedure enables each group member to play a truly participating role. During this time, there is no discussion permitted regarding form, format, or meaning of a participant's response.

5. Clarify the meaning of the responses.

Take time to inquire as to whether or not each response is clearly understood. Allow participants time to discuss what they meant by a particular response, the logic behind it, and even its relative importance. However, this is not the time for argumentation and lobbying. The group leader must direct the proceedings so that only clarification takes place.

6. Conduct a preliminary vote.

From the original listing of responses on the blackboard or flip-chart, participants are directed to select a stated number of the items they consider the most important (e.g., out of the original 20 responses, each participant is to select and rank seven of them). This is accomplished by writing each one of the statements selected on a separate card first, and then rank-ordering them (in the example provided, seven points would be assigned to the most important item, and one would be assigned to the least important). Delbecq et al. point[s] out that, as a rule of thumb, group members can prioritize only five to nine items with some degree of reliability. Participants are asked to list the item number along with the statement in the upper left-hand portion of the card. When all the participants have accomplished this for the seven statements they have selected, they are then asked to rank the cards by placing the rank number in the lower right-hand portion of the card and underlining it. On the blackboard or flip-chart, the group leader then records the rankings assigned to the statement selected by each participant and sums up the votes after all participants have contributed their rankings. The item with the largest numerical total represents the top priority issue. In usual instances, this is as far as one need go in the process. However, it can be extended to include the following steps, in order to assure accuracy.

7. Discuss the preliminary vote.

It is important to discuss the various explanations related to the voting patterns. Discussion regarding the high vote-getters and low vote-getters may be of value. It may also be useful to redefine the meaning of selected items, to be certain that all participants are clear on their meaning.

8. Conduct a final vote.

For this step, two procedures can be used: (a) as followed in the preliminary vote, select a stated number of the most important items, and then rank-order them; or (b) select a stated number of the most important items, and then rate them. To describe this second procedure in more detail, if there are seven major items selected, each one of them could be rated on a scale of zero (not important) up to ten (very important). This procedure then provides insight regarding the actual magnitude of differences between the major items.

9. Calculate the total vote.

Remembering that there may be several groups of six to seven members each which are going through this process (e.g., there may be 12 groups working simultaneously or at varied time intervals), it is important to calculate a grand total vote. First, the items from all of the groups are arranged into similar categorical areas (if at all possible), and then the numbers from rank-ordering or rating are added together in each categorical area. For example, if three items from group one, two items from group two and four items from group three relate to health problems with rodent infestation, the total value (from ranking or rating) is calcualted for all nine items. The resulting value is then listed for the categorical need area of "Health problems related to rodent infestation." As the total votes are calculated for each categorical area, it will be realized that they can be placed in descending order. The categorical area with the largest number is considered to be of the highest priority.[13]

The Delphi Method

Another method useful at this stage, especially if face-to-face meetings are impractical, is the Delphi method. In this method a series of questionnaires is mailed to a small number of experts, opinion leaders, or informants. Differences of opinion among various key people can be resolved by the planner without forcing confrontation. Linstone and Turoff develop the method most fully, but Gilmore provides a brief description of the method as it applies to health education:

1. Define the issue.

A planning committee should develop a clear and concise statement as to the central issue to be addressed. For example: "The need to identify the top priority barriers related to rural health care delivery in Minnesota and Wisconsin."

2. Establish who the participants will be.

Individuals must be selected who are knowledgeable about the subject at hand. They must also be able to handle the written format which will be used. Since the process is accomplished via mailed materials, there can be a wide dispersal of those involved. Using the mail system also prevents those participants with high professional positions from influencing others, since they will not meet face-to-face, as in the nominal group process. Usually from 15 to 30 participants nominated by the planning committee can provide the needed input.

3. Develop the first questionnaire.

This is the first mailing which goes out to the participants after they have agreed to become involved in the process. An introduction should clarify the central issue for the participant. Instructions should then be given for him to respond to an open-ended format. For example, the statement could be made: "Please indicate on the enclosed form those items which you feel are top priority barriers to rural health care delivery in Minnesota and Wisconsin." Also, it is important to give the participants approximately a two-week deadline in which to return the first questionnaire. Upon the return of all questionnaires, the items are collated into appropriate categories representative of the items' meanings.

4. Develop the second questionnaire.

Taking the resulting categories, these are listed on the second questionnaire with response sections next to them on the sheet. While any necessary information can be requested in the response sections, two frequently used formats include priority voting and comments. Thus, if there were 20 categories of barriers which resulted from the first questionnaire, the participants could be asked to rank the top seven, as well as add comments about any of the 20 categories. Again, a deadline for the return of the questionnaires should be set.

    A. *Instructions:* "As you will note, the responses to the first questionnaire resulted in 123 items, which have been compiled into 20 categories. Please select the seven most important barriers and rank them: 7 = most important; 1 = least important in this group of seven barriers. Also, please add your comments about any of the 20 items."

    B. *Barriers* (list of 20 items)

	Vote	*Comment*
1. Inaccessibility	____	_____
2. Inadequate transportation	____	_____
20. Family problems	____	_____

5. Develop the third questionnaire.

The values which were assigned to each category on the second questionnaire are added together and entitled the "initial vote total." Also, a summary of the participants' comments is prepared for each category receiving votes. This information is used to develop the third questionnaire which also provides a space for "final votes." Upon the return of this questionnaire, the totals for the "final vote" sections should be calculated, leading to the arrangement of the categories in descending priority order.

  A. *Instructions:* "Below you can see the results of the second questionnaire. Please cast your final vote for the seven most important barriers (7 = most important)."

  B. *Barriers* (list of 20 items)

	Initial vote	Final vote	Previous comments
1. Inaccessibility	73	____	Always important
2. Inadequate transportation	67	____	Affects many
20. Family problems	8	____	Not major

6. Final considerations.

It is quite possible to construct a fourth questionnaire whenever the material needs to be more finely analyzed. Whether or not such a questionnaire is generated, a final report of the last questionnaire results should be sent to participants.

  Some of the unique advantages of this process become quite obvious. Researchers are able to work with a variety of target group representatives, as long as they are considered to be knowledgeable about the issue of concern. Since it is mailed, the format makes possible a wide geographical outreach. It also means that large numbers can be handled. However, it should be kept in mind that having more than 30 respondents may not result in enhanced results. During the process, the participants remain anonymous, thus protecting the generated ideas from the influences of group conformity, prestige, power, and politics.[14]

  Small-scale telephone or mailed surveys to members of a target population can be economical and effective in estimating the prevalence and intensity of suspected concerns but are not efficient at the exploratory stage.[15]

The Continuum Approach

Another general class of methods is associated with helping people clarify their own values.[16] One method appropriate to this stage of planning is an adaptation of the continuum approach described by Kreuter.[17] In this strategy participants are asked to indicate the level of quality of life for themselves or their community by placing an X on a quality of life continuum with values ranging from "poor" to "optimum" (fig. 2.2a). Once the participant has placed an X on the continuum, he or she is told to divide the continuum

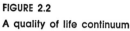

FIGURE 2.2
A quality of life continuum

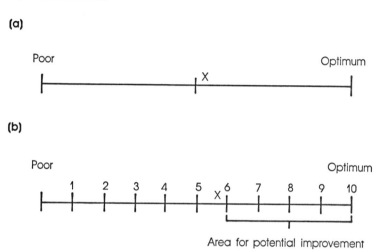

into ten equal units, numbering them from 1 to 10 from left to right (fig. 2.2*b*).

The assumption is that the distance between the X and 10 is representative of the area for potential improvement in perceived quality of life. Participants are then asked why they perceive the quality of life of their community to be 5 or 6 or anything less than 10. As an answer to that question, they are asked to list several conditions that they believe stand as barriers to an improvement in the quality of life. Thus, specific data on perceived problems and needs in their community are generated. An advantage of this method is that it is appropriate for use in small and large groups as well as in one-to-one settings.

Using Public Service Data

Data on perceived needs and problems are more readily available than one might realize. For example, a sometimes overlooked but rich source for this kind of data is the broadcasting media. Television and radio broadcasters are required by the Federal Communication Commission to ascertain community needs and concerns regularly and to offer public service programming to address those problems. In Baltimore, Maryland, for instance, a coalition of radio and television broadcasters employs an independent group to conduct public opinion surveys periodically to identify the needs and problems of the Baltimore area as seen through the eyes of those who work and live there. In addition, the coalition conducts monthly meetings with local government, religious, and neighborhood leaders to get their ideas about existing community problems. Most broadcasters across the nation have similar programs and will share their data when they are asked to do so.

INTERPRETING THE DATA

Once gathered, the quality of life indicators (both the objective data and the perceived needs) should be studied to identify those standing as the most formidable barriers to a desired quality of life. Some of the objective indicators can be calculated in terms of frequency counts, incidence rates, rates under treatment, utilization rates, and frequency distributions. Those that can be calculated can be compared with previous measures of the same indicators to ascertain trends or changes in problems. This kind of analysis allows a health education planner to see if a given problem is mushrooming, gradually disappearing, or remaining static. A quality of life assessment can not be made solely on the basis of statistical analysis, however. Ultimately the major resource for health education planners during this important first step of the diagnostic process is critical observation and good professional judgment. The final determination of quality of life concerns must be made by means of careful consideration of the available evidence, including the sentiments of the members of the community—the patients, students, workers, or citizens—who are the intended benefactors.

"Taking the temperature and pulse" of the community as we suggest in phase 1 is a consciousness-raising activity for the health educator, for the others in his or her organization who will be engaged in the overall health education program, and for the patients, students, workers, or citizens. It reveals the reasons for educational interventions.

But is it realistic in most situations for the health education planner to expect to be able to do a quality of life assessment before planning his or her programs? Although the procedure may not always be systematic and well developed, and although it may not be started and finished by the same person, most programs are planned and delivered to meet a need that has caused sufficient concern to merit the call for educational attention. For example, alcohol and drug "units" or classes in school health education programs can trace their origin to the public's perception of the ill effects of alcohol and drug abuse on society.[18] National and international population and family planning education programs have been and continue to be funded in the expectation that they might help reduce the social maladies that so often accompany overpopulation and problem pregnancies.[19] Self-care health education efforts are currently offered with the hope that reductions in medical costs and time lost due to illness and increased self-esteem and personal control will be, along with better health; program outcomes.[20] Indeed, it is probably safe to say that most health education programs with any significant support from the general public are addressing health problems that have been identified as potentially detrimental to quality of life.[21]

What has triggered the relatively recent interest by some corporations in occupational health education? Is it corporate benevolence or regulatory constraints imposed on industry because society has deemed intolerable the problems it creates? To the executive it probably makes good business sense to support programs that will make workers more productive, be absent less often, have fewer accidents, and reduce their claims on disability and health insurance. It is clear in this circumstance that health education has benefits outweighing its costs.[22] Such benefits may be perceived first by workers, then by society through its elected or appointed representatives; but ultimately employers, too, will recognize such benefits, in the form of improved public relations and greater worker satisfaction and productivity.

SIX OBJECTIVES OF PHASE I

It is not our intention to encourage planners in this phase to gather extensive statistical data that are not already available (although sample surveys may be appropriate and feasible).[23] The objectives of this phase can be achieved by interpreting and supplementing information from existing records, files, publications on social indicators, and informal interviews and discussions with leaders, key informants, and representative members of the target community.[24] In summary, the objectives are six:

1. to *determine* the subjective concerns with quality of life in the target population
2. to *verify* and clarify these concerns with analyses of existing social indicators and data available from newspaper files, census reports and vital records, and special surveys conducted by radio and television stations and marketing and social service agencies
3. to *document* the status of the target community in relation to those priority concerns for which there is a health component or cause
4. to *make explicit* the rationale for the selection of priority problems
5. to use the documentation and rationale to *justify* the further expenditure of health education resources on the selected social problems
6. ultimately, to use the documentation and rationale as the bases on which to *evaluate* the program in cost-benefit terms

STEPPING IN

As we have noted, many who conduct health education activities, particularly those in clinical, school, and industrial settings, will be given the task of developing a program based on a quality of life assessment (or something similar) that has already been done by someone else. In fact, an epidemiological diagnosis (discussed in the next chapter) may also have been completed. Because this situation is common in health education, especially in patient education and in some community health agencies, those who find themselves in it should make a special effort to become familiar with the information used by others in the assessment process. Such a review provides the crucial foundation information needed to keep perspective on the health education goal.

SUMMARY

The identification and analysis of the social problems of a target population is a necessary first step in thorough health education planning. Health is not an ultimate value in itself except as it relates to social benefits or quality of life. It is important to study the inseparable relationship between health problems and social problems or quality of life. Several specific techniques that the health educator can use in gathering information about social problems and perceived quality of life for a given population are described.

EXERCISES

1.   How did (or would)* you involve the members of the population you selected in exercise 3, chapter 1 in identifying their quality of life concerns? Justify your methods in terms of their feasibility and appropriateness for the population you are helping.

2.   How did (or would) you verify the subjective data gathered in exercise 1 with objective data on social problems or quality of life concerns?

3.   Display and discuss your real or hypothetical data* as a quality of life diagnosis, justifying your selection of social, economic, or health problems for priority attention on the basis of their perceived and objective importance in the lives of your population.

---

*It is recommended that these exercises be carried out with a real population accessible to the student or practitioner, but if this is impractical the exercises can best be followed with a well-described hypothetical population using actual Census data and health information from similar populations.

3

Epidemiological Diagnosis: Assessing Etiologies

IN THE PRECEDING CHAPTER the ultimate mission of health education programs was fixed as improvement in the quality of life. Agreement on aspects of life perceived to have negative effects on its quality is the correct starting point in justifying and planning health programs, educational programs, and, especially, health education programs. In this chapter, we shall explore the second step in the PRECEDE framework: the identification of the health problems associated with an unsatisfactory quality of life.

IDENTIFYING HEALTH PROBLEMS

Of the multitude of problems causing concern with quality of life, health educators must, of course, direct their efforts toward the solution of health

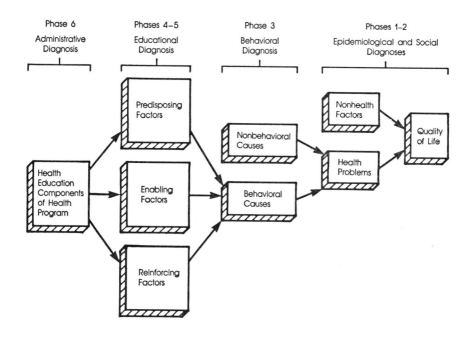

Phase 6	Phases 4–5	Phase 3	Phases 1–2
Administrative Diagnosis	Educational Diagnosis	Behavioral Diagnosis	Epidemiological and Social Diagnoses

Predisposing Factors

Nonhealth Factors

Quality of Life

Nonbehavioral Causes

Health Problems

Health Education Components of Health Program

Enabling Factors

Behavioral Causes

Reinforcing Factors

problems. Epidemiologic data show the incidence, prevalence, and distribution of relevant health problems and can suggest the importance of these problems in relation to quality of life. These data, supplemented by theoretical and scientific literature on the natural course and etiology of the problems and information about the activities of the community and local agencies, help health educators set priorities in planning. Epidemiologic information also guides the formulation of specific program objectives.

Social problems as such are rarely the immediate focus of a health education endeavor. (Unemployment, for example, might be ameliorated by health education, but a specific program in health education will seldom tackle more than the health aspects of unemployment.) Instead, health educators almost invariably invest their professional energies in improving the health status of certain groups or communities. Health outcomes constitute the most concrete long-range goals of most health education programs, even if those goals are explicitly justified in terms of the potential they have for contributing to the social or economic good. There are two principal approaches to identifying health problems susceptible to intervention.

The Reductionist Approach

One approach consists of deriving health problems *exclusively* from an existing statement of social problems and an inventory of all the determinants of the social problems. In the PRECEDE framework (fig. 1.3) social diagnosis, or quality of life assessment, is the initial step. In everyday practice, however, most health professionals must start their planning with existing data already reduced by someone else to a categorically specified health problem such as diabetes or skin cancer. Rarely is one in a position to survey the overall quality of life in a community as a formal precursor to specifying which health problems deserve attention. Such surveys are routinely conducted, however, by various public, private, and voluntary agencies with mandates other than health, and they can be used to identify social problems affecting a particular population. Using data on unemployment, substandard housing, illiteracy, welfare, isolation, or other social problems, the health professional can analyze the rates of occurrence or distributions of health problems in a target population. Using epidemiologic knowledge and methods, he or she can then recommend priorities for programs directed at health problems and for other programs directed at nonhealth factors that contribute to the social problems of greatest concern.

A review of the scientific and professional literature is also a prerequisite to a professional response to social problems. The relationship between health problems and the social problem of poverty (for example) is analyzed in a number of works.[1]

Figure 3.1 suggests generally how poverty can be separated into contributing health-related and nonhealth-related factors as a basis for program planning according to the PRECEDE framework. The distribution and severity of health problems must, of course, be determined for each local community. Members of a rural community might suffer to a greater degree from parasitic infections, anemia, malnutrition, and serious maternal and child health problems than people who live in an inner-city ghetto, where alcoholism, mental illness, and excess fertility might predominate. One responsibility of the health professional is to interpret local data in light of medical and epidemiological knowledge concerning cause-effect relationships and the natural history and distribution of health problems.

Nonhealth factors contributing to the social problem also will vary depending on the makeup of the target population and its location. Migrant workers and their families might suffer from poor access to organized social

FIGURE 3.1

Health and nonhealth factors contributing to poverty

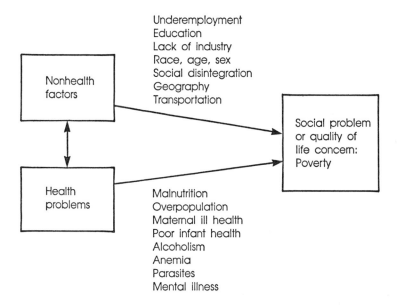

support systems such as education and welfare. Poor roads or geographic isolation might figure in poverty status, as might lack of jobs. Also, racial or ethnic minority status more often than not contributes to social and health problems. Except on their own time health professionals usually are not expected (and sometimes are not allowed) to intervene in nonhealth matters. Nonetheless, it helps to be aware of the potential effect of socioeconomic factors on the solution of a health problem. Say, for instance, that the health educator thinks it appropriate to tackle malnutrition problems. Unless the target population can have access to gardens, to greater financial resources to invest in food, or to food supplements, they may have difficulty changing their diets.

Such could have been the case in the remarkable early years of the Mound Bayou Community Health Center in Mississippi, opened in the late 1960s. In the Mound Bayou community poor nutrition was a major problem, which the health center leadership thought could be best attacked by encouraging community members to plant home gardens (and by, supplementally, providing information on nutritional preparation of food). It had to overcome bureaucratic resistance to this approach, but improved nutritional status was the result. Health workers are often not able to use the approaches that seem most direct, but they can initiate cooperative efforts with other community agencies, and they can refer patients to other resources. In coping with social problems health workers clearly must take into account relationships between health and nonhealth factors. Otherwise, they run the risk of addressing forces rendered trivial or insurmountable by the context.

In the reductionist approach, then, one works from the broader social problem toward a diagnosis of its health components or causes. "Reduction" is the first step in epidemiological diagnosis—assessing the relative importance of various causes or etiologies—when the social problem has been identified (as in chap. 2) but the causes of the problem have not been clearly delineated. When, as often happens, so many causes demand attention that health workers are in danger of frittering away their efforts, the reductionist approach can be used to arrive at the manageable, important few by means of methods described later in this chapter.

The Expansionist Approach

Health professionals are usually trapped. They are assigned to work on a specific health problem (such as hypertension, tuberculosis, or obesity) with a known target population. Someone else has already reduced the ultimate problem to a specified health problem. Because of the scarcity of resources, however, it is important to weigh the importance of the assigned health problems against that of others to make sure that health education is focused on those the reduction of which will yield the greatest benefit.

Within the context of a limited mandate, then, it is useful to survey the scene from a larger perspective. For a national perspective two excellent documents are *Forward Plan for Health* (dealing with conditions in the United States) and Lalonde's *A New Perspective on the Health of Canadians.* Both describe major health problems and their distribution in relation to their burden on society. Another source, *Source Book of Health Insurance Data,* issued yearly by the Health Insurance Institute,* provides the latest statistics relating specific health conditions to quality of life or economic factors (table 3.1).

Such data give the "trapped" health educator an idea of the relative impact of his or her assigned problem. Consider the following example. A health educator has been asked to develop a health and safety education program for the control of injuries to women over the age of forty-five working in a large industry. He or she checks the national figures (as shown in table 3.1), which reveal that (1) noninjury problems account for a larger number of workdays lost by women in this age group and (2) work-loss days from injuries are more prevalent in other ages and in males. Even without support from local data, which are not often available, the health educator is in a

---

*1850 K Street N.W., Washington, D.C. 20006.

TABLE 3.1

Workdays lost due to acute conditions: United States, 1976

Acute conditions	Number of work-loss days (000,000)			Work-loss days per employed person		
	All ages 17 and over	Ages 17–44	Age 45 and over	All ages 17 and over	Ages 17–44	Age 45 and over
MALE						
All acute conditions	186	124	62	3.6	3.7	3.4
Infective and parasitic diseases	12	9	*	0.2	0.3	*
Respiratory conditions	77	49	27	1.5	1.5	1.5
Digestive system conditions	10	6	4	0.2	0.2	0.2
Injuries	62	45	17	1.2	1.3	0.9
All other acute conditions	25	14	11	0.5	0.4	0.6
FEMALE						
All acute conditions	140	100	40	4.0	4.3	3.5
Infective and parasitic diseases	15	10	5	0.4	0.4	0.4
Respiratory conditions	67	47	20	1.9	2.0	1.7
Digestive system conditions	6	5	*	0.2	0.2	*
Injuries	24	16	8	0.7	0.7	0.7
All other acute conditions	28	22	6	0.8	0.9	0.5

SOURCES: *National Health Survey* and National Center for Health Statistics.

NOTE: The data refer to the civilian, noninstitutional population. An acute condition is one that lasted less than three months and that involved either medical attention or restricted activity. A "work-loss day" is a day on which a currently employed person, 17 years of age and over, did not work at least half of his or her normal workday because of a specific illness or injury. In some cases the sum of the items does not equal the total shown, because of rounding.

*Figures do not meet standards of reliability or precision.

strong position to argue for shifting attention to a different health problem, to women in a different age group, or to men in this or another age group.

The expansionist approach is particularly useful when the assigned problem has been oversimplified. Suppose a newspaper article announces an alarming comparison between the local infant mortality rate and the state-wide rate. A statement on the newspaper's editorial page denounces the quality of infant care in local hospitals, and the city council calls for a corrective program. Faced with this situation, a health education planner in a maternal and child health program might analyze the following information:

- A two-county rural area, populated mainly by a low-income minority agricultural group, has unacceptable rates of maternal and infant mortality.
- The maternal death rate is 65.5/100,000 compared to the state rate of 18.4/100,000.
- The infant mortality rate is 34.5/1,000 live births compared to the state rate of 21.0/1,000.
- The fetal death ratio remains at 24.9/1,000 live births in spite of an overall decline in the state rate to 14.6.
- Problems identified include high incidence of prematurity, low infant birth weights, a pattern of fetal distress and respiratory distress at delivery, plus observed failure to thrive. The visiting nurse service also reports prevalence of anemia, high incidence of GI infection and respiratory diseases.
- Many mothers are at risk because of age—a disproportionate number between fourteen and seventeen—poor nutrition, lack of medical care, multiple pregnancies, as well as toxemias of pregnancy.
- Childhood accidents are common; children look undernourished; they report for school with handicapping conditions and no immunizations.[2]

According to this information, the chief cause of the relatively high infant mortality rate in the area is not deficiencies in the quality of infant care in local hospitals; the corrective program should not consist of buying new, improved hospital equipment. By expanding his or her understanding of the problem and seeing the alarming statistics in the broader context of relationships between health and social problems, the health educator can help the community address the problem more comprehensively and productively through prevention and health promotion.

This example illustrates two other points. First, the relationship of health problems to quality of life can be quickly discerned. High rates of adolescent pregnancy likely lead at least to school absenteeism if not to dropping out. And to a greater proportion of single-parent homes, which often are in lower income brackets and in need of proportionately greater social services, may also result. Handicapped children require special treatment, which has implications for distribution of a community's resources for day care, teachers, and family welfare.

Second, the example suggests the vital importance of developing data for significant subgroups, in this population, the low-income, minority, agriculture group; teenage girls; and their infants. In other populations data might reveal higher prevalence of hypertension among black males or of lung cancer among white middle-aged males. Without such data, it would be impossible for the trapped health professional to know which subpopulations should receive special attention and which health problems deserve higher priority than the assigned one.

DESCRIBING HEALTH PROBLEMS

It is important to describe health problems in detail. Going through the process serves three principal functions: (1) It helps establish relationships between the health problem, other health conditions, and quality of life; (2) it leads to fuller understanding of the various dimensions of the health problems, which in turn gives a basis for setting priorities and serves as a guide for concentrating program development and resources; and (3) it can make possible a clear allocation of responsibilities among collaborating professionals, agencies, or departments. These points should be clearer as we further explore how to describe health problems fully.

Establishing the Dimensions

The classic indicators of health problems are mortality, morbidity, fertility, and disability (or the 5 Ds: death, disability, disease, discomfort, and dissatisfaction). Comparative data on these indicators are available from a variety of sources, such as the National Center for Health Statistics, other agencies of the Department of Health, Education and Welfare (or the ministry of health in other countries), local and state health departments, the Bureau of the Census, professional journals and associations, the World Health Organization, and local, regional, and state planning agencies.[3] It is helpful to know whether the rates in the target population are significantly better or worse than rates in *comparable* populations.

A New Perspective on the Health of Canadians gives data on trends in one classic indicator, mortality. Of the 157,300 deaths in Canada in 1971, nearly half (75,200) were people under seventy years of age and were considered "early deaths." The leading contributors to premature deaths in those over thirty-five were found to be cardiovascular diseases.

As one indicator of the burden of cardiovascular diseases, hospitalization rates were also inspected. It was found (for 1970) that diseases of the cardiovascular system accounted for 7,600,000 hospital days (20 percent of the total). This figure can be contrasted to that for accidents, 3,100,000 hospital days.[4]

As the planner gathers detailed comparative information on incidence, prevalence, distribution, intensity, and duration of the problem, he or she will become aware of the aspects of the problem that have potential for change.

Of the diseases of the cardiovascular system, let's take hypertension as an example. Suppose a member of the staff of a city health department has been asked to coordinate planning for a hypertension screening program. Table 3.2 shows national data on hypertension for the years 1971–74. Incidence is highest among blacks and older age groups. Also of interest to the planner are the rates per 100 hypertensives of people with previously undiagnosed hypertension. Pursuing the matter, the planner discovers that the relationship between race, education, and hypertension has been studied by the Hypertension Detection and Follow-Up Program. Its work suggests that education does not fully account for differences in rates of hypertension between black and white populations (table 3.3).[5] In the event there are no data of this sort available for a target population, the health planner must extrapolate regional or national data (table 3.4).

The data in table 3.4 confirm that hypertension is a serious health problem in the community (X), particularly in the black population that the health department predominantly serves. Furthermore, low-income populations generally have less access to health care, which further complicates the problem, given the critical role of prolonged treatment in controlling high blood pressure.

At this point the planner has narrowed the problem by locating the subpopulations in which the health problem is most prevalent. The epidemiological diagnosis has served its first purpose, which is to focus the attention of the planner on the aspect of the problem or part of the population where intervention can be most useful.

The planner can gain another useful perspective on hypertension as a health problem by looking at the more specific information available in community surveys. In 1974, 21,268 people in Washington County, Maryland, for example, had their blood pressure checked. Of those, 10 percent were found to have untreated high blood pressure; another 13 percent were already under treatment for hypertension.[6] In table 3.5 the data from Washington County are compared to those from three other, earlier, surveys, and the percentage of hypertensive patients in different phases of treatment and control is indicated. Screening for elevated blood pressure appears to be much less a problem in Washington County than convincing individuals with suspected hypertension to stay on medical treatment. A planner working in Washington County would focus the health program on treating detected cases rather than on screening for new cases. In Alameda County, on the other hand, the percentage of treated cases in which high blood pressure was

TABLE 3.2

Prevalence rates of definite hypertension among whites and blacks 18–74 years, by age, sex, and percentage with this condition not previously diagnosed: United States, 1971–74

| | Rates per 100 population | | | |
| | Whites | | Blacks | |
	Men	Women	Men	Women
Definite hypertension*				
TOTAL	18.5	15.7	27.8	28.6
18–24 years	4.9	1.4	4.6	2.9
25–34 years	8.2	3.7	17.7	10.2
35–44 years	17.3	10.1	38.2	28.3
45–54 years	25.8	18.9	36.8	50.9
55–64 years	31.1	31.7	49.9	54.5
65–74 years	35.3	42.3	50.1	58.8
Definite hypertension not previously diagnosed†				
TOTAL	64.5	48.2	54.9	41.2
18–24 years	67.0	66.4	90.4	62.6
25–34 years	71.1	65.0	52.0	57.0
35–44 years	66.8	57.5	38.2	40.8
45–54 years	64.3	58.9	71.8	44.3
55–64 years	62.1	39.2	48.9	33.0
65–74 years·	61.9	41.2	51.0	39.1

SOURCE: National Center for Health Statistics, *Blood Pressure of Persons 6–74 years of age in the United States,* NCHS Advance Data no. 1, October 18, 1976.

NOTE: An estimated 19.4 million white persons at ages 18–74 years out of 113.6 million and 3.7 million Negro persons at ages 18–74 years out of 13.0 million have definite hypertension as defined in this table.

*Systolic blood pressure of at least 160 mm Hg or diastolic blood pressure of at least 95 mm Hg.

†Percentage of persons with definite hypertension, as defined in this table, who have never been told by their doctors that they have high blood pressure.

controlled was high (63.2 percent), but the percentage on medication (35.7 percent) was low relative to Washington County, so more screening would have been an appropriate emphasis.[7]

TABLE 3.3

Prevalence of hypertension at first screening, by age, level of education, and 151,668 adults screened for hypertension: Fourteen U.S. communities, 1973–74

Age and race	Percentage hypertensive, by years of education completed				
	<10	10–11	High school graduate	Some college	College graduate
30–39 years					
Whites	8.9	9.8	7.1	6.8	6.2
Blacks	26.6	23.9	18.9	15.3	13.7
40–49 years					
Whites	16.6	16.7	14.7	14.8	13.8
Blacks	41.2	34.7	30.9	30.0	25.2
50–59 years					
Whites	22.9	23.8	22.7	22.0	20.3
Blacks	47.2	44.5	41.1	40.2	37.9
60–69 years					
Whites	30.4	28.8	28.2	27.5	25.5
Blacks	50.4	46.4	47.8	42.9	50.8

SOURCE: Hypertension Detection and Follow-up Program Cooperation Group: "Race, education and prevalence of hypertension." *American Journal of Epidemiology* 106 (1971): 351–61.

NOTE: Hypertension = average diastolic pressure of 95 mm Hg and/or reporting current use of antihypertensive medication.

Sometimes the planner may want or even need to conduct his or her own survey to verify the extent of the problem in the target population. Valid data may not be available, or it may be necessary to use a survey as a means of stimulating community participation in the project. The extent of available resources (human and fiscal) and time will influence the decision on whether to conduct a survey.

Setting Priorities

Full description of the health problem (or problems) and how it is manifested in the target population is essential to the setting of sound priorities.[8] Should there be several problems, the task of selecting one from among them calls for answers to the following questions:

TABLE 3.4
Estimated number of adults in city x with elevated blood pressure

	White			Nonwhite			Total
	18–44 years	45–64 years	65+	18–44 years	45–64 years	65+	
A　Population (from Census)	142,080	98,619	71,300	174,758	77,389	27,849	591,995
B　Prevalence of high blood pressure*	7.5/100	26.8/100	39.3/100	16.5/100	48.3/100	55.1/100	
$\frac{A \times B}{100}$　Number estimated to have high blood pressure*	10,656	26,430	28,021	28,835	37,379	15,345	146,666

*Prevalence rates based on regional data similar to the data shown in table 3.2 and derived from the same source.

TABLE 3.5
Estimated reservoir of undetected and untreated individuals with elevated blood pressure

Characteristics of populations surveyed	Baldwin County, Ga. 1962 N = 3,084	National Health Survey 1960–62 N = 6,627	Alameda County, Ca. 1966 N = 2,495	Washington County, Md. 1974 N = 21,268
Percentage with elevated blood pressure 160 systolic and over and/or 95 diastolic and over	17.5	15.2	13.0	16.9
Percentage on medication for hypertension*	6.0	6.5	5.9	12.7
Percentage with elevated blood pressure on medication for hypertension†	18.3	23.2	16.9	5.6
Percentage of total hypertensive population on medication	29.7	35.7	35.7	52.8
Percentage of total hypertensive population "under control"	14.0	16.3	22.6	29.4
Percentage of persons on medication "under control"	47.0	45.6	63.2	55.6

*In the Washington County survey, this percentage may include persons with treatment other than specific medication. Total hypertensive population equals those with blood pressure 160 systolic and/or 95 mm Hg diastolic at the time of survey plus those on medication for hypertension with survey pressures below those levels.

†In determining percentages in Alameda County, a systolic level of 165 (not 160) was used.

1. Which problem has the greatest impact in terms of: death, days lost from work, rehabilitation costs, disability (temporary and permanent), family disorganization, and cost to communities and agencies to repair damage or recover losses?
2. Are subpopulations, such as children or mothers, at special risk?
3. Which problems do "state of the art," available technology, and the agency's mandate and capacity make most susceptible to intervention?
4. Which problem is not being addressed by other agencies in the community? Is there a need that is being neglected?
5. Which problem, when appropriately addressed, has the greatest potential for an attractive yield—in improved health status, economic savings or other benefits to the community, and positive visibility for the agency?
6. Is one or more of the health problems highly ranked as a regional or national priority? Health systems agencies are developing priorities among health problems, for instance, based on extensive reviews of epidemiologic data from their areas.

Elaborating on the scope and impact of the health problems helps the planner get a clear focus on the problems and the strategies to be used in attacking them. This procedure may also help in deciding whether a program is to be preventive, curative, rehabilitative, or some combination of these perspectives. Consider the complex problem of motor vehicle accidents, succinctly outlined in *Forward Plan for Health.* [9] Prevention efforts might consist of trying to reduce drunken driving or increase use of seat belts in combination with consistent enforcement of the 55-mile-per-hour speed limit. The emphasis of a curative program would be on immediate emergency medical services (including transportation of accident victims to the appropriate facility). A rehabilitative effort would deal with disabilities resulting from accidents, increasing the number of victims who regain productive lives and the speed with which they do so. Epidemiologic information may suggest which facet or facets of the problem will (or *will not*) yield to intervention; and it will suggest which focus—preventive, curative, or rehabilitative—should be paramount.

Ensuring Knowledgeable Cooperation

Detailing the health problem helps to harmonize the activities of the various individuals and groups involved in the program. Health education usually is part of a larger endeavor, one engaging a variety of disciplines if not also several units within an agency. Hospital-based health programs, for example, might function across inpatient and outpatient units and social service and nutrition departments. Programs based in a health department will often deploy staff from various personal-health-services units as well as from environmental protection units and other sections. The more heterogeneity there is among participants (and perspectives), the greater the utility of sharply delineated statements of the problem. All participants in the activity need to share a full understanding of it. Understanding is further facilitated when program goals and subobjectives are thoroughly spelled out.

Restricted Objectives

It is not unusual for health workers to be associated with programs having restricted target populations and program objectives. Family planning, diabetes, maternity, hypertension, smoking, and dental programs are just a few examples. Epidemiologic and medical data can provide cues for couching program objectives for such programs in terms of reducing certain risk factors associated with the health problem (weight control for hypertensives; smoking cessation for patients with heart diseases; absence of sugar or acetone in urine of diabetic patients). Health education directed toward reducing risk factors in a designated subgroup can be as appropriate and may be more feasible than that directed toward long-range reduction in incidence or prevalence of particular illnesses.[10]

DEVELOPING COHERENT PROGRAM OBJECTIVES

When the health problem has been specifically defined, the next step is to develop the program objectives. This vital phase in program planning is frequently treated superficially, with unfortunate consequences in terms of program implementation and evaluation. Objectives are crucial; they form a fulcrum, converting diagnostic data into program direction. Objectives should be cast in the "language" of epidemiologic and medical data, answering the questions: *Who* will be the recipients of the program? *What* benefit should they receive? *How much* of that benefit should they receive, *by when*, or for how long? Consider the maternal and child health data presented on page fifty-four. One objective built on those diagnostic data, consonant with the mission or resources of the agency, was:

- Reduction of maternal mortality rate within counties A and B by 10 percent within the first two years and an additional 15 percent the next three years, continuing until the state average is reached.

The target population (*who*) is demographically implied (pregnant women) and geographically explicit (within counties A and B). The *what is* reduced maternal mortality. *How much* benefit is to be achieved *by when* is stated in stages: a 10 percent reduction in two years, a 25 percent reduction in a total of five years, and the program is to continue until the state average rate is achieved. (Note that the average rate for the state will probably go down concurrently, so the program has tackled a moving target.)[11]

In developing program objectives, the planner should be sure that: (1) progress in meeting objectives can be measured; (2) individual objectives are based on relevant, reasonably accurate data; and (3) objectives are in harmony across topics as well as across levels.

For objectives to be in harmony across topics means that objectives dealing with various aspects of a health problem (e.g., objectives in a maternity program to improve nutrition, prenatal appointment compliance, weight and blood pressure control, and percentage of hospital deliveries) should be consistent with each other. Objectives should also be coherent across levels, with objectives becoming successively, level by level, more refined and more explicit. In the usual language of health planners, goals are considered to be more general than objectives. For example, the maternal and child health program objective just presented is in reality part of a three-tier hierarchy of concordant objectives consisting of an overall program goal, a set of more specific program objectives, and a number of even more specific objectives stated in behavioral terms:

- *Program goal*
  The survival rate of mothers, infants, and children will be raised through raising the quality of prenatal care and promoting the optimal growth and development of children.

- *Program objectives*
  Maternal mortality rate within counties A and B will be reduced by 10 percent within the first two years and an additional 15 percent the next three years, with reductions continuing until the state average rate is reached.

- Infant mortality rate will be reduced to the state average within ten years. Perinatal mortality rate will be reduced from 49 . . . Fetal death will be reduced . . .

- *Behavioral objectives*
  In the two counties, 1,850 women under age forty who have had two or more pregnancies will have two general health checkups the first year of the program.

- Eighty percent of pregnancies in this group will be detected within the first trimester, and prenatal care with special diets will be instituted.

■ Ninety-five percent of the pregnant women will be delivered by qualified medical personnel in obstetric facilities during the first year of the program.

Note that the objectives in this example, ranging from the broadest statement of program mission to the most immediate and precise target, are coherent. Achievement of each of the more specific and more immediate objectives will contribute in a causal sense to the achievement of the more general and more distant objectives and goals. Behavioral objectives are the subject of the next chapter.

SUMMARY

This chapter highlights the relationship between health problems and social problems. Health professionals usually do not deal directly with social problems per se, but they will find critical analysis of the relationship between each health problem addressed by a program and the quality of life to be instructive. Health problems should be described in detail using data from local, regional, state, and national sources interpreted against a background of current epidemiological knowledge as reflected in the literature. Particular attention must be directed toward identifying existing data on who is most affected (age, sex, race, residence), the ways in which they are affected (mortality, disability, signs, symptoms), and the most likely routes to improvement (impact of immunizations, treatment regimens, environmental alterations, behavioral changes). This information helps set program priorities for health problems that are both important and changeable. Program priorities are expressed as program objectives by specifying *who* will benefit *how much* of *what* outcome by *when*. A thorough epidemiological diagnosis is basic to the next phase of the PRECEDE framework (which is identifying the behavioral components of the health problem.)

EXERCISES

1. List the health problems related to the quality of life concerns identified in your population in exercise 3, chapter 2.

2. Rate (low, medium, high) each health problem in the inventory according to (a) its relative importance in affecting the quality of life concerns, (b) its potential for change.

3. Discuss the reasons for your ratings of health problems as having high priority in exercise 2a in terms of their prevalence, incidence, cost, virulence, intensity, or other relevant dimensions. Extrapolate from national, state, or regional data when local data are not available.

4. Cite the evidence supporting your ratings of health problems in exercise 2b. Refer to the success of other programs and/or to the availability of medical or other technology to control or reduce the high-priority health problems you have selected.

5. Write a program objective for the highest-priority health problem, indicating *who* will show *how much* of *what* improvement by *when.*

4

Behavioral Diagnosis: Assessing Health Actions

WE HAVE DESCRIBED HEALTH EDUCATION as an activity designed to facilitate voluntary adaptations of *behavior* conducive to health. That interpretation of purpose leads from the identification of health problems or risks, as discussed in chapter 3, to the third phase of the PRECEDE process: behavioral diagnosis. Simply stated, *behavioral diagnosis* is the systematic identification of health practices that appear to be causally linked to the health problem or problems identified in the epidemiological diagnosis.

WHY AN EMPHASIS ON BEHAVIOR?

Regardless of what they do, all health professionals have a common long-term goal: to improve the health and quality of life of the people they serve.

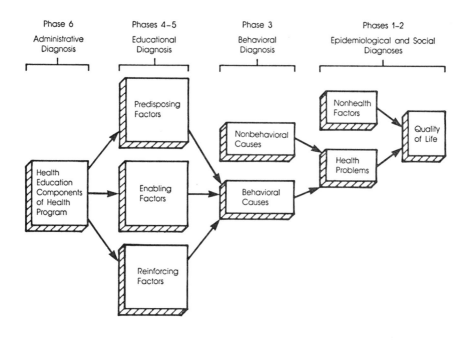

Phase 6	Phases 4–5	Phase 3	Phases 1–2
Administrative Diagnosis	Educational Diagnosis	Behavioral Diagnosis	Epidemiological and Social Diagnoses

No matter where, how, and by whom it is offered, health education is a process related to health decisions and practices. Knowledge, values, perceptions, and motivation are, of course, causes of behavior, but the linkage between them and desirable health practices is a matter of probability. In the final analysis, health education programs are effective only to the extent that they influence the health practices found in research to be causally related to the desired health outcomes. The first task in behavioral diagnosis, then, is to establish cause-and-effect relationships between behavior and health. In the PRECEDE framework, "behavioral problems" refers to the behaviors believed to cause health problems for the people *for whom the educational intervention is intended*. After considerable analysis, target behaviors are selected and the approach to changing them stated in terms of behavioral objectives. Behavioral objectives are the means by which program objectives and program goals are achieved.

FIGURE 4.1
Behavioral and nonbehavioral causes of health problems

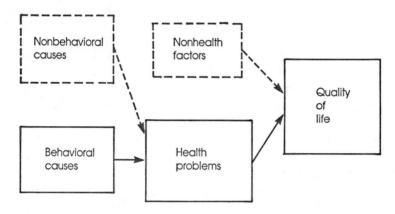

Health problems have both behavioral and nonbehavioral causes (fig. 4.1). Although behavioral diagnosis is directed toward specific behaviors, careful consideration must also be given to nonbehavioral causes. Nonbehavioral causes are personal and environmental factors that can contribute to health problems *but that are not controlled by the behavior* of the target population. Such causes include: genetic predisposition, age, gender, existing disease, physical and mental impairment, climate, work place, and residence. We will discuss some of these in the next chapter, in which we examine the causes of behavior. Here they are significant insofar as they contribute to health problems. The health practitioner who takes the contribution of nonbehavioral factors to health problems into account will be better able to

1. maintain perspective on the multiple determinants of the health problem being attacked
2. identify factors for which strategies other than health education (such as political or environmental) may be developed and concurrently used
3. select and rank the behaviors that will be the focus of the program

Health education is sometimes accused of "blaming the victim," because it appears to place all the responsibility for protection of health on the individuals whose health is threatened. Recognizing the nonbehavioral causes of health problems acknowledges that there are other threats to health besides the behavior of the victim.

Most of the nonbehavioral causes of health problems are either environmental (air, water, roads, fluoridation, etc.) or technological (adequacy of medical care, facilities). Such causes can be influenced by behavior of the pub-

FIGURE 4.2

Three ways behavior can influence health

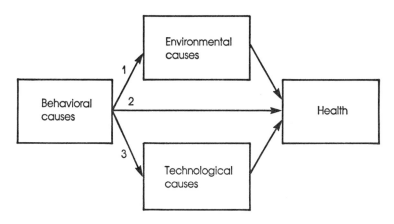

lic or the victims, especially through collective action. Communities, neighborhoods, or special-interest groups such as self-help groups can organize, vote, boycott, lobby, or otherwise support or prevent certain environmental and technological changes. Thus, behavior can influence health in three ways, one direct and two indirect, as shown in figure 4.2.

Failure to identify nonbehavioral factors and recognize how they might affect outcomes can cloud the results of an otherwise sound program. Consider the following example. The West Virginia chapter of the American Lung Association wants to sponsor a health education program for a population of coal miners in two counties in northern West Virginia. Epidemiological data clearly suggest that the incidence of lung disease in miners in this area is greater than it is in other areas of the state, a situation that the association would like to change. If the health problem is studied in terms of behavioral and nonbehavioral causes, certain epidemiological questions will surface: Do all miners get lung disease? Who gets lung disease and who doesn't? Are all mine workers male? Do those who have lung disease also have a family history of the disease? Answers to such questions, directed at nonbehavioral factors (such as age, sex, family history), identify the high-risk groups. Once the high-risk group (or groups) has been identified, one asks questions about behavior. Is there a higher incidence of the disease in smokers than in nonsmokers? Do those who work at different levels of the mines or at different jobs show differing incidences of disease? What is the relative risk by specific age group for those who started smoking at different ages? These kinds of questions can help the practitioner select the behaviors that will be the subject of the behavioral objectives and the focus of the intervention.

Health education efforts do not have as much impact as they should when the behavioral objectives are vague and grossly conceived. Given the scarcity of health education resources, vagueness is an ill-afforded luxury. When the target behavior is "intangible" and can not be measured, it is usually because the behavioral components of the health problem have not been sufficiently delineated. Behavioral objectives are sometimes stated in terms as vague as "improve health habits" and "increase the use of health services." Educational effort aimed at such diffuse targets is likely to be scattered, with the result that too little education is directed at any one behavior to make a difference.

THE FIVE BASIC STEPS IN BEHAVIORAL DIAGNOSIS

Behavioral diagnosis can be accomplished by means of five basic steps. To get a feel for the five steps, consider a sample problem.

Suppose a state health department has just completed a quality of life assessment and epidemiological diagnosis. On the basis of the findings, the director wants to allocate some of her resources to the health problem of cardiovascular disease. She gives a planning team the task of developing a demonstration health education project that will reduce the incidence of cardiovascular disease in the state. Epidemiological diagnosis has suggested that the intervention should consist of a primary prevention program aimed at youth and young adults who are asymptomatic. The behavioral diagnosis is next.

Step 1: Differentiating Between Behavioral and Nonbehavioral Causes of the Health Problem

The planner's first step is to differentiate between the behavioral and nonbehavioral causes of the health problem, and he or she begins, in the case of cardiovascular disease, by listing the known risk factors for the disease.

smoking	heavy alcohol consumption
gender	diabetes
sedentary life-style	obesity
stress	age
high serum cholesterol	family history of disease
high blood pressure	high fatty-acid intake

Which of these factors are behavioral and which are not? Some are easy to classify. Smoking, heavy alcohol consumption, and high fatty-acid intake are *clearly* behavioral; whereas gender, age, family history of heart disease, and diabetes are nonbehavioral. High serum cholesterol, obesity, high blood pressure, sedentary life-style, and stress, while not strictly behavioral factors, are closely tied to behavior. High blood pressure, serum cholesterol, and obesity are linked to eating; and sedentary life-style and, in part, stress, are associated with inactivity and lack of exercise. Analysis will show which factors are only apparently nonbehavioral.

Step 2: Developing an Inventory of Behaviors

Once the behavioral and nonbehavioral factors have been listed, the list of behavioral factors should be refined. The procedure is twofold.

- *a.* Identify the behaviors associated with preventing the health problem and state them in terms of actions to be taken.
- *b.* Identify the treatment procedures of the health problem in sequential order. What are the steps that people have to go through to "comply" with a recommended method of prevention or treatment? Each step is a behavior.

It is important for the planner to keep in mind that the major aim of step 2 is to generate a list of highly specific behaviors that can be used as the basis for specifying the behavioral objectives of the program.

Table 4.1 shows such a list. Notice that many of the behaviors appear as both preventive behaviors and treatment behaviors. This is not at all unusual, and the information is valuable. If a single behavioral problem (smoking) appears in both parts of the inventory, a change in the behavior (stopping smoking) increases the probability of positive health gains whether the level of prevention is primary or secondary. Primary prevention consists of actions taken in the absence of signs or symptoms. Secondary prevention is directed toward early detection and treatment.

This list, even though it consists of several distinct behaviors, is crude and nonspecific. Some of the behaviors listed actually comprise several specific behaviors. The behavior maintaining or attaining desirable weight, for example, is the result of other behaviors such as buying low-calorie foods, cooking foods with less fat, serving smaller portions, eating fewer portions, minimizing desserts, and substituting fresh fruits for desserts with high sugar content. For the purposes of this and the following two steps, the list is specific enough.

When behaviors are to be translated into behavioral objectives, however, it is necessary to break them down into the actual steps that people will go through in achieving each behavioral goal.

TABLE 4.1
Inventory of behaviors

Preventive behaviors

    1. Maintain or attain desirable weight.
    2. Stop smoking or don't start.
    3. Stop heavy or abusive drinking or don't start.
    4. Continue or begin regular exercise.
    5. Avoid excessive, constant stress and/or do relaxation exercises.
    6. Participate in high blood pressure screening programs.

Treatment behaviors

    1. Make informed decisions regarding medication, surgery, and so forth.
    2. Take prescribed medication.
    3. Maintain or attain desirable weight.
    4. Stop smoking.
    5. Stop heavy or abusive drinking.
    6. Continue or begin regular exercise.
    7. Avoid excessive, constant stress and/or do relaxation exercises.

One approach to analyzing behavior in more specific terms is to develop a flow chart of causation or transition from beginning to end of a behavioral process or event. For example, the behavior of taking prescribed medication (table 4.1) requires several behavioral processes: seeking medical care, obtaining a prescription, and seeing that the prescription is adapted to changes in blood pressure. It can be sabotaged at many points along the way, for example, when the hypertensive patient fails to keep medical appointments where prescriptions might be renewed or adapted. The "broken appointment cycle"[1] can be analyzed as a series of causes and effects (fig. 4.3). This level of specificity makes it possible to isolate concrete behavioral events from nonbehavioral factors in such a way as to ensure that interventions—educational and administrative—are highly targeted.[2] Other approaches to analyzing behavior are discussed in the *Journal of Applied Behavioral Analysis* and the *Journal of Behavioral Medicine*.

Step 3: Rating Behaviors in Terms of Importance

With an extensive list of behaviors in hand, the next step is to reduce the list to a manageable length by establishing which behaviors are the most important. The following guidelines are designed to help in that task. Behaviors should be considered most important when (1) data are available clearly linking the

FIGURE 4.3
The broken appointment cycle

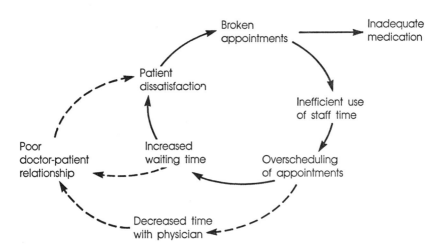

behavior to the health problem and (2) they occur frequently. Behaviors are considered less important when (1) they are tenuously or very indirectly related to a health problem and desired outcome and (2) they are rare. Behaviors can also be considered important if a strong theoretical case can be made for their being causally related to a health problem. In lieu of adequate data, such a case may be developed from a thorough review of the literature. The stronger the rationale, the greater the probability that the behavior selected for intervention will be the right one.

Which behaviors from the sample problem will receive top priority? Ratings are presented in table 4.2. Keep in mind that the program is to have an impact on the incidence of cardiovascular disease and that the focus is to be on primary prevention.

Step 4: Rating Behaviors in Terms of Changeability

The next step in a behavioral diagnosis is rating behaviors in terms of changeability. How changeable are the selected behaviors? A behavior may be extremely important to a health problem, but it may also be just short of impossible to change through health education. For example, more than one authority has made the claim that excessive stress is associated with cardiovascular disease.[3] Before a change in stress could be noted, however, conditions in the work place and at home would likely have to be altered. How feasible is that for a health education program?

TABLE 4.2
Rating the importance of behaviors associated with cardiovascular disease

Important	*Basis for rating behavior*
Smoking	Very strong association; high incidence
Eating foods with high fatty-acid content	Strong association; high incidence
Overeating	Moderate association; high incidence
Lack of exercise	Moderate association; high incidence
Not relaxing	Moderate association; high incidence
Not (less) important	*Basis for rating behavior*
Not monitoring blood pressure	Not related to the
Not adhering to medical regimen	desired outcome of the
Making uninformed decision about treatment matters	program: primary prevention

Judgments about changeability must also include careful consideration of the time factor. How much time is there to show change? The more deeply rooted and widespread the behavior, the more important time is as a factor.

Again, there are guidelines that can help the planner ascertain potential for changeability. High changeability is probable when behaviors (1) are still in the developmental stages or have only recently been established, (2) are only superficially tied to established cultural patterns or life-styles, and (3) have been successfully changed in other programs. Behaviors have low changeability when they (1) have long been established, (2) are deeply rooted in cultural patterns or life-styles, and (3) have not been changed in previous attempts. These guidelines suggest as a corollary that the earlier the intervention occurs in the growth and development of the subjects, the greater the probability for change.

In another approach to the assessment of changeability, the characteristics of the behavior that make it more or less easy to adopt are analyzed, using criteria from the literature on adoption of innovations.[4] However, this method, called the attribute method (illustrated table 4.3) should be used only for behaviors that can not be ruled out using the cruder but more direct and efficient criteria suggested in the previous paragraph. Note that a total changeability score for each behavior can be obtained simply by adding horizontally across the columns, scoring 1 for a plus sign and −1 for a minus sign.

TABLE 4.3
Relative changeability of various preventive behaviors, based on perceived attributes of the behavior

Health behavior	Relevance	Social approval	Advantage	Complexity	Compatibility with values, experiences, and needs	Divisibility or trialability	Observability
1. Quitting smoking	+	+	+	−	−	+	+
2. Controlling weight	+	+	+	−	−	+	+
3. Controlling blood pressure	+	0	−	−	−	+	−
Taking medication	+	0	−	−	−	+	−
Maintaining low sodium diet	+	−	−	−	−	+	−
4. Maintaining low cholesterol diet	+	0	+	−	−	+	−
5. Exercising	+	+	−	−	+	+	+
6. Having preventive medical examinations	+	0	−	+	+	−	+

SOURCE: Adapted from L. W. Green, "Diffusion and Adoption of Innovations Related to Cardiovascular Risk Behavior in the Public," in *Applying Behavioral Sciences to Cardiovascular Risk*, eds. A. Enelow and J. B. Henderson (New York: American Heart Association, 1975).

NOTE: + = positive; 0 = neutral or ambivalent; − = negative.

TABLE 4.4
Rating the changeability of behaviors associated with cardiovascular disease

Changeable	Basis for rating behavior
None	
Not (less) changeable	
Smoking	Since youth will make up our target population, it is reasonable to assume that many of the pertinent behaviors are in the developmental or early adoption stages, suggesting the possibility of high changeability. Nevertheless, the degree to which the behaviors are rooted in life-style is varied, and previous attempts to change them have not been uniformly successful.
Eating foods with high fatty-acid content	
Overeating	
Lack of exercise	
Not relaxing	

Note: Behaviors that were rated unimportant in table 4.2 have been eliminated from this rating.

The score could be adjusted, recognizing that not all the criteria are of equal importance in determining changeability of the behavior. The more important criteria could be given greater weight if their relative importance could be estimated.

By testing behaviors for changeability, we come one step closer to an informal decision on which behaviors should be slated for intervention. Table 4.4 shows the changeability ratings. None of the behaviors has been given a high-changeability rating. Although arguments can be made against such a conclusion, findings in the literature on primary prevention of cardiovascular disease are too inconsistent to place any of the behaviors with confidence in the high-changeability category.[5]

Step 5: Choosing Behavioral Targets

With the behaviors ranked in terms of importance and changeability, the planner is ready to select the behavior or behaviors that will be the focus of the

FIGURE 4.4
Matrix of health behaviors

	Important	Not (less) important
Changeable	1. High priority for program focus	3. Low priority except to demonstrate change for "political" purposes
Not (less) Changeable	2. Priority for innovative program; evaluation crucial	4. No program

educational intervention. To facilitate that selection, we recommend that the results of the importance and changeability ratings be arranged in a simple fourfold table (fig. 4.4).

Depending on the program objectives, the behaviors selected to be the subject of the behavioral objectives will more than likely come from quadrants 1 and 2. Evaluation is crucial when there is uncertainty whether change will occur. Behaviors found in quadrant 3 will be unlikely candidates except when there is a political need to document change, as is the case when administrators or advisory committees need "evidence" of achievement. When such a need exists, the behaviors should be given only temporary priority. Sometimes there will not be any behaviors in quadrant 1 (as in the sample problem). If there are none but the health problem identified is urgent, an extensive educational and behavioral research and evaluation effort is justified. Frequently, this is how agencies and foundations determine their own research priorities.

Figure 4.5 shows how the behaviors generated in the sample problem would be placed in a matrix. There are no behaviors in quadrant 1, but quadrant 2 carries six behaviors that are important factors in preventing cardiovascular disease. For none of these behaviors, however, is there conclusive evidence of potential for significant change in response to educational interventions. During the planning meeting to select the behaviors that will be the focus of the program, one of the team members cautions against choosing several behaviors, thereby spreading limited resources too thinly. After discussion, it is agreed that *one* behavior must be chosen. Another member of

FIGURE 4.5
Matrix of health behaviors—sample problem

	Important	Not (less) important
Changeable	1. None	3. None
Not (less) Changeable	2. Smoking Eating foods with high fatty-acid content Overeating Lack of exercise Not relaxing	4. None

the planning team mentions an article by Borhani, a thorough and scholarly critique on the primary prevention of coronary heart disease. The article is distributed and reviewed by all team members. Two of the author's conclusions are particularly significant in the context:

> Until we learn more about the role of the lipid hypothesis and control of hypertension in prevention of coronary heart disease, one of the most rewarding activities in today's medical practice could be advice on smoking, because if even a relatively small reduction in the death rate from coronary heart disease were to result a great number of lives would be saved. Because it is much easier not to start smoking than to stop, our clinical efforts toward prevention should be directed primarily toward the pediatric age group, especially since it takes a few years for the beneficial effects to appear.[6]

Since there is some evidence concerning successful smoking programs, the planning team decides to narrow its focus to a single behavior: smoking.

STATING BEHAVIORAL OBJECTIVES

Once the target health behavior (or behaviors) has been identified, the planner is prepared to take the final step: stating behavioral objectives. As suggested earlier in this chapter, if the behavioral objectives are vague and loosely defined, educational efforts are likely to be scattered rather than focused. Where behavioral change is desirable, possible, and appropriate, utmost care should be given to stating objectives precisely. Each behavioral objective should answer the question: *Who* is expected to achieve *how much* of *what* behavior by *when*?

- *Who*—the people expected to change
- *What*—the action or change in behavior or health practice to be achieved
- *How much*—the extent of the condition to be achieved
- *When*—the time in which the change is expected to occur

What might be a behavioral objective for the sample problem? The target behavior is smoking. The planning team has determined that the program should be conducted in county A because it is demographically representative of the majority of the state and similar to several counties in adjoining states. The "who" will consist of all residents aged fifteen to twenty-five in county A. The "what" will be a reduction in the incidence of cigarette smoking. "How much" will be established as 20 percent, adjusted for the present national data, which show a steady decline in smoking prevalence.* The "when" will be by the time of the proposed follow-up evaluation, two years after the program is initiated. Concisely stated, then, the behavioral objective will read: Young adults aged fifteen to twenty-five in county A will show a 20 percent reduction in incidence of cigarette smoking within two years of program implementation.

SUMMARY

As a result of working through the first phases of the PRECEDE framework (chaps. 2 and 3), three foundations are laid:

1. Advanced thinking about or *planning* of health education programs should begin with an assessment of the quality of life of the population to be served by the health education program.
2. Given the results of an assessment of the quality of life problems of a target community, an epidemiological diagnosis can identify specific health problems that stand as barriers to quality of life.
3. Program objectives should be based on findings from quality of life assessments and the epidemiological diagnosis.

---

*"How much" can be an individual behavioral objective such as reducing each smoker's consumption of cigarettes by 20 percent or a program objective of reducing overall consumption by 20 percent.

In this chapter in showing how to identify the most fruitful behavioral targets for a health education program, we take the next step in the PRECEDE framework. If health educators are to be accountable for improvements in or maintenance of health, then the limited educational resources available for this purpose need to be concentrated on the health practices most likely to contribute to health improvement or maintenance.

Each health problem identified in the epidemiological diagnosis requires a separate behavioral diagnosis. Each behavior identified in the behavioral diagnosis requires a separate educational diagnosis. Failure to be parsimonious in the selection of problems, then, leads to the multiplication of educational diagnoses required (and, concomitantly, to the diffusion of resources). The use of rigorous criteria and the application of critical judgment in the epidemiological diagnosis makes the work of behavioral diagnosis easier. Severely testing health behaviors according to their importance and changeability will save considerable effort in the upcoming educational diagnoses. And, finally, the concise statement of behavioral objectives will lead to greater specificity in program development and will simplify the evaluation process.

EXERCISES

1. In relation to the highest-priority health problem identified in your program objective in exercise 5, chapter 3, list the specific behaviors in your population that might be causally related to the achievement of that objective.

2. Rate (low, medium, high) each behavior in your inventory according to its (a) prevalence, (b) epidemiological or causal importance, and (c) changeability.

3. Provide or cite objective evidence supporting your ratings in exercise 2. Extrapolate or interpolate from national, state, or regional data when local data are not available or cite data from similar populations or studies elsewhere.

4. Write a behavioral objective for your population (*who*) showing what percentage (*how much*) will exhibit the behavior or change the behavior (*what*) by a given date or amount of time from the beginning of a program (by *when*).

5

Educational Diagnosis: Assessing Causes of Health Behavior

THUS FAR, IN GOING THROUGH THE PROCESS of planning a health education program, we have shown how social, epidemiological, and behavioral diagnoses can be made. In the next phase of the PRECEDE framework, the educational diagnosis, the behaviors identified as linked to the health problem or problems of greatest concern in a population are differentiated according to what causes them. The educational diagnosis is an indispensable part of determining how best to initiate the process of behavior change.

For convenience, the factors causing health behavior are seen to be of three distinct kinds: predisposing, enabling, and reinforcing. Each kind has a different type of influence on behavior.

Predisposing factors are factors antecedent to behavior that provide the rationale or motivation for the behavior. Included are knowledge, attitudes, beliefs, and values. *Enabling factors* are factors antecedent to behavior that allow a motivation or aspiration to be realized. Included are personal skills and

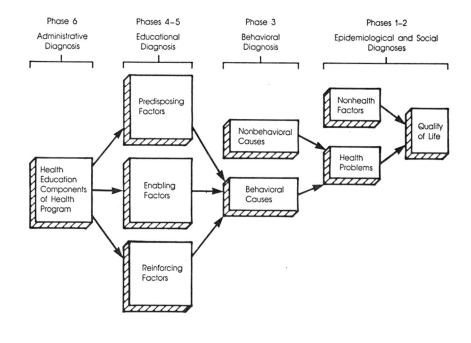

Phase 6	Phases 4–5	Phase 3	Phases 1–2
Administrative Diagnosis	Educational Diagnosis	Behavioral Diagnosis	Epidemiological and Social Diagnoses

resources as well as community resources. *Reinforcing factors* are factors subsequent to behavior that provide the continuing reward, incentive, or punishment for a behavior and contribute to its persistence or extinction. Included are social as well as physical benefits and tangible as well as imagined or vicarious rewards.

Any given health behavior may be seen as a function of the collective influence of these three factors. The notion of collective causation is particularly important because behavior is a multifaceted phenomenon. Any plan to change behavior must take into account not one but several influencing factors. Said another way, programs in which health information is disseminated without concurrent recognition of the influence of enabling and reinforcing factors will most likely fail to affect behavior.

Note that the constellation of predisposing, reinforcing, and enabling factors is not thought to form an all-inclusive causal model of health behavior change. The main utility of the model is that it makes it possible to sort the determinants of behavior change that are most responsive to health education into categories convenient for planning.

To say that behavior is a complicated phenomenon is an understatement. Countless theories have been developed attempting to explain human behavior, yet no single theoretical model has been universally accepted. Models are constantly being modified in response to new situations. Croog and Peters note precisely that circumstance in their study of factors related to smoking patterns:

> From the many conceptual models which have been developed as a means of explaining preventive health behavior, some common themes emerge which provide useful leads for examining long-term change and stability in smoking behavior. As there is no comprehensive and generally accepted single model, we have felt free to draw upon particular elements in the literature relevant to our data. [1]

Our approach in identifying predisposing, enabling, and reinforcing factors as determinants of behavior change is similar. Our rationale is based on several common theoretical themes that seem to be especially applicable and appropriate to health education.

Figure 5.1 focuses attention on some assumptions about the causal relationships among factors to be considered in the educational diagnosis. The order of causation, as indicated by numbers, is normally expected to be (1) an initial motivation to act, (2) a deployment of resources to enable the action, (3) a reaction to the behavior from someone else, resulting in (4) the reinforcement and strengthening of the behavior or the punishment and discouragement of the behavior. Finally, (5) reinforcement or punishment of the behavior affects the predisposing factors, as do the enabling factors (6).

PREDISPOSING FACTORS

Predisposing factors, which include knowledge, attitudes, beliefs, values, and perceptions, relate to the motivation of an individual or group to act. In a general sense, we can think of predisposing factors as the "personal" preferences that an individual or group brings to an educational experience. These preferences may either support or inhibit health behavior; in any case, they are influential. Although a variety of demographic factors such as socioeconomic status, age, gender, and present family size are also important as predisposing factors, they are beyond the direct influence of a health education program.

FIGURE 5.1

Three categories of factors contributing to health behavior

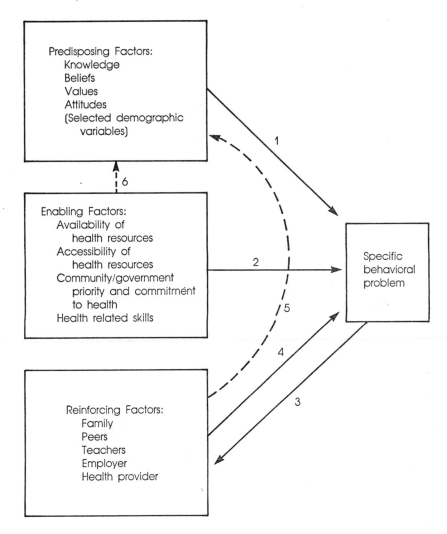

NOTE: Solid lines imply contributing influence, and dotted lines imply secondary effects.
Numerals indicate the approximate order in which the actions usually occur.

Knowledge

An increase in knowledge does not always cause behavior to change, but positive associations between the two variables have been demonstrated in the early work of Cartwright,[2] the recent Stanford Three-Community Study,[3] and in numerous studies conducted in the interim. Health knowledge of some kind is probably necessary before a personal health action will occur, but the desired health action will probably not occur unless a person receives a cue strong enough to motivate him or her to act on the knowledge he or she has.[4]

Consider, for example, the case of school health education. It is frequently justified by reference to the simple, commonsense notion that knowledge is the best road to wisdom and to action. Proponents of the opposing position argue that the goals of knowledge and wisdom are too "soft" and intangible to be used as criteria for program effectiveness in school health education. Furthermore, they state that contemporary students are disenchanted and bored by facts. We disagree. Students are not turned off by facts; they are turned off by moralization, superficial coverage of subject matter, and tedious methods of presentation. By misinterpreting the cause of dissatisfaction, some health teachers may be abandoning information and facts in favor of affective exercises and armchair moralization about how one should behave to be healthy.

It is as ludicrous to say that knowledge makes no difference as it is to say that it makes all the difference. The appropriate perspective to keep is an intermediate one, that knowledge is a necessary but not sufficient factor in changing health behavior.

Beliefs, Values, and Attitudes

Beliefs, values, and attitudes are independent constructs, yet the differences between them are often fine and complex. Inasmuch as this book is directed to the practitioner rather than the researcher, we will forgo the technicalities and examine these factors in a practical way, trusting that those interested in more detailed analysis will look further in the theoretical research literature.[5]

Beliefs   A *belief* is a conviction that a phenomenon or object is true or real. *Faith, trust,* and *truth* are words used to express or imply belief. Health-oriented belief statements include such statements as: "I don't believe that medication can work"; "If this diet won't work for him, it sure isn't going to work for me"; "Exercise won't make any difference"; "When your time is up, your time is up, and there's nothing you can do about it." If beliefs such as these are strongly held, to what extent will they interfere with good health? Can they be changed? Will changes facilitate health-promoting behavior?

The Health Belief Model, notably employed by Hochbaum, Rosenstock, Leventhal, Kegeles, Kirscht, and Becker, attempts to explain and predict health-related behavior in terms of certain belief patterns.[6] The model is based on the following sequence of events. For behavior change to occur,

1. The person must believe that his or her health is in jeopardy.
2. The person must perceive the potential seriousness of the condition in terms of pain or discomfort, time lost from work, economic difficulties, and so forth.
3. On assessing the circumstances, the person must believe that benefits stemming from the healthy behavior outweigh the costs and are indeed possible and within his or her grasp.
4. There must be a "cue to action" or a precipitating force that makes the person feel the need to take action.

This last point is perhaps fundamental to the entire model. Health education can provide the cue to action if the predisposing factors represented by the health beliefs are correctly diagnosed.

Values   Consider this brief exchange between two people.

He: Did I hear you say that you are going to try skydiving?

She: Absolutely not!

He: Why not?

She: Because I value my life, that's why not!

He: Do you also value your health?

She: Of course I do.

He: Then why do you smoke cigarettes?

She: Because I enjoy smoking and it helps me relax.

He: If that's the case, can you honestly say that you really value your life?

She: Sure I can. It's not that I don't value my life and health but that I value other things too, among them the pleasure of smoking. What's wrong with that?

It goes without saying that personal values are inseparably linked to choices of behavior. In the scenario above, the person who values life, health, and cigarettes too, is revealing a conflict of values. For values to be in conflict is not at all uncommon. According to the former Canadian Minister of National Health and Welfare, "Most Canadians by far prefer good health to illness, and a long life to a short one but, while individuals are prepared to sacrifice a certain amount of immediate pleasure in order to stay healthy, they are not prepared to forgo all self-indulgence nor to tolerate all inconvenience in the interest of preventing illness."[7]

Conflicts in health-related values represent one of the important dilemmas and challenges for health education practitioners. Values theory and values-clarification teaching strategies are well represented in the education and health education literature and merit the utmost consideration in the health education planning process.[8] Helping people to sort through conflicts in their health-related values is an important health education technique.

Attitudes *Attitude* is one of the vaguest yet most frequently used words in the behavioral sciences lexicon. To keep matters short and simple, we offer two definitions that in combination cover the principal elements of *attitude*. Mucchielli describes *attitude* as "a tendency of mind or of relatively constant feeling toward a certain category of objects, persons or situations."[9] Kirscht indicates that *attitudes* represent a collection of beliefs that always includes an evaluative aspect;[10] that is, attitudes can always be assessed in terms of good and bad or positive and negative.

Health educators should keep in mind the two key concepts: Attitude is a rather *constant* feeling that is *directed toward an object* (be it a person, an action, or an idea); and inherent in the structure of an attitude is *evaluation,* a good-bad dimension. We can gain further understanding of the structure of attitude by examining one of the techniques frequently used to measure attitudes: the semantic differential.[11] This technique calls for responses to be made to concepts by means of making a mark on a continuum between antonyms. Suppose we want to measure the attitudes expressed by the woman in the dialogue toward skydiving and cigarette smoking. Having heard her conversation with the man, we already have an idea about what her attitudes are, but let's measure them just the same.

Concept: Skydiving

good   :__ :__ :__ :__ :__ : X :__ : bad

pretty   :__ :__ :__ :__ :__ : X :__ : ugly

happy   :__ :__ :__ :__ : X :__ :__ : sad

Concept: Cigarette smoking

good   :__ : X :__ :__ :__ :__ :__ : bad

pretty   :__ :__ : X :__ :__ :__ :__ : ugly

happy   : X :__ :__ :__ :__ :__ :__ : sad

From the conversation and from what we can see now in her response, it is clear that her attitudes toward both skydiving and smoking are constant.

Since they are constant, they are probably also strong. We can also see the woman's evaluation (in terms of good and bad) of the concepts. Neutral responses can be registered on the continuum, and the woman didn't make any.

The relationships between behavior and constructs such as attitudes, beliefs, and values are not completely understood, but the evidence that they exist is ample. Analysis will show, for example, that attitudes are to some degree the determinants, components, and consequences of behavior. This alone is sufficient reason to continue to be concerned with attitudes, beliefs, and values as predisposing factors.

ENABLING FACTORS

Enabling factors are the skills and resources necessary to perform a health behavior. Such resources include health care facilities, personnel, schools, outreach clinics or any similar resource. Enabling factors also pertain to the accessibility of various resources. Cost, distance, available transportation, hours open for use, and so forth, are enabling factors of this sort. Finally, personal health "skills" such as those discussed in the literature on self-care and school health education are considered enabling factors. [12]

When we use the term *skills* here, we are referring to a person's ability to perform the tasks that constitute the desirable behavior. Skills can range from the appropriate use of relaxation techniques and physical exercise to the use of the variety of medical instruments and diagnostic procedures frequently required in self-care programs. Assessing the extent to which members of the target population possess enabling skills can give the planner valuable insight into possible program components. Failure to consider the impact of enabling factors on the achievement of behavioral goals can lead to serious practical problems.

Suppose a well-intended educational effort has been successful in raising the motivation of members of a target group to make greater use of medical services in their area. However, the health care providers in the area were not consulted. If they had been, it would have been found that existing facilities were already overcrowded and that providers felt overworked and not at all willing to take on more work without an expansion of facilities and additional personnel. What will the outcome likely be? Participants in the program will not get the service that they need and were promised; they may become discouraged and feel as if they have been "let down" again; health care providers may become angry with and alienated from health education efforts because they were not considered and were made to look bad for not delivering services that had been promised. As we have emphasized throughout this book, a health behavior has many causes, so unidimensional efforts to affect behavior rarely, if ever, produce the desired results.

In a position paper on the effects of enabling factors, Milio contends that the health behavior of a population may be limited by the degree to which health resources are made available and accessible by health organizations: "Organizational behavior . . . sets the range of options available to individuals for their personal choice-making."[13]

REINFORCING FACTORS

Reinforcing factors are those that determine whether health actions are supported. The source of reinforcement will, of course, vary depending on the objectives and type of program. In occupational health education programs, for example, reinforcement may be provided by co-workers, supervisors, union leadership, and family. In patient education settings, reinforcement may come from nurses, physicians, fellow patients, and, again, the family. Whether the reinforcement is positive or negative will depend on the attitudes and behavior of significant people, some of whom will be more influential than others in affecting behavior. For example, in a high school health education program, where reinforcement may come from peers, teachers, school administrators, and parents, which group is likely to have the most influence? While there are no absolute answers to that question, research in adolescent behavior does indicate that adolescent drug-taking behavior is most influenced by approval from friends,[14] especially a best friend.[15] Further, parental attitudes, beliefs, and practices, especially those of the mother, are extremely influential in affecting the health status of their children.[16] Which people are significant may vary not only according to the setting but perhaps by growth and development stages as well. Program planners must carefully assess reinforcing factors to make sure that program participants have maximum opportunities for supportive feedback during the behavior change process.

SPECIFYING AND SELECTING FACTORS
DETERMINING BEHAVIOR

The core of the educational diagnosis is selecting from among the reinforcing, predisposing, and enabling factors those that if modified will help to bring about the behavior desired. There are three basic steps in this process: (1) identifying and sorting factors into the three categories; (2) setting priorities among categories; and (3) establishing priorities within the categories. Specific factors selected by this process form the basis for learning objectives, which will then lead to the selection of materials and methods for program implementation (chap. 6). If the program is well designed and carefully carried out, the probability is high that the learning objectives will be met and the target behaviors modified.[17]

Identifying and Sorting

The list of factors generated for each behavior should be as comprehensive as possible. In this way, the planner may be able to avoid overlooking a crucial item, a pitfall when his or her attention is diverted by each item as it is listed. Both informal and formal methods can be used to develop the list.

Informal methods   The team assigned the responsibility for designing the plan usually has made some educated guesses and hypotheses about the reasons why people do or do not behave in the desired manner. It is crucial that members of the group at risk (the consumers or target population) become involved in the planning again at this point. Their information and insight on the group's present behaviors, attitudes, beliefs, values, and other potential barriers to reaching the stated objectives are most relevant. Intensive interviews, informal group discussions, nominal groups, focus groups, panels, and questionnaires about services provide useful data.[18]

The same methods of eliciting information can be used with staff who will be involved in the delivery of the services and people in agencies providing related services. They might suggest causes of behavior ranging from ignorance and negative attitudes to unrecognized effects of agency or community policies and operations. Systematic recording of the data will make them useful and retrievable.

Brainstorming and nominal group process are useful techniques for generating data on barriers to behavioral change.[19] A vital step in PRECEDE is the sorting of factors according to whether they are seen as having negative or positive effects. The negative effects must be overcome, and the positive effects can be built on and strengthened.

The planner must be critical in accepting the ideas of health care providers on predisposing factors affecting patients or clients. Some providers may interpret undesirable behavior different from the expectations of the middle-class professional as stemming from laziness, apathy, or ignorance. Generalizations of this sort do little to explain the behavior at issue. "Blaming the victim" may arise out of misunderstanding, poor communication, or rationalization. The system may be at fault, rather than the patient.[20]

Formal methods   A search through the relevant literature can yield information on cultural and social attitudes and descriptions of studies defining the impact of specific factors on health-related behavior.[21] Such a search may also yield items that can be used on survey questionnaires or as part of record-keeping systems (see chap. 8).

Checklists and questionnaires are structured ways of collecting and organizing information from important individuals and groups. These can be used to measure knowledge, attitudes, and beliefs as well as perceptions of services.

Directories of available community resources are often compiled by planning agencies. These directories are particularly helpful when enabling factors are being examined. Utilization data from health care organizations and attendance records from agencies are also available.[22]

If the planners have trouble deciding whether a factor is predisposing, enabling, or reinforcing, they should list it in whichever categories might apply. The three categories are not mutually exclusive; a factor can appropriately be placed in more than one column. A family may be predisposed to dieting, for example, and reinforce (negatively or positively) that behavior once it has been undertaken.

Later in the planning process, specific educational activities and messages will be related to these factors. Then the category of the factor will make a difference. For example, messages and learning opportunities provided at the predisposing point will be different according to whether a family is seen as an important factor in creating motivation or it is seen as an important source of reinforcement.

A list at this point might look something like the one in table 5.1, which shows both positive and negative factors related to reducing the sequelae of streptococcal throat infections in a preschool population. At the end of this chapter we shall show how to convert some of these factors into learning objectives, which are statements of the immediate goals of a health education program. Learning objectives must be achieved in order to obtain voluntary behavioral changes, which are the intermediate goals of the program. The behavioral objectives must be achieved if there are to be health improvements, which are the ultimate goals of the program.

Setting Priorities Among Categories

There is no way that all the causes in a complete inventory for several behaviors can be tackled simultaneously. Decisions about which factors are to be attacked first and in what order are therefore necessary.

One possible basis for establishing priorities among the three kinds of factors is developmental. People will not adopt a set of behaviors to reduce a health risk if they are not aware that there is a risk. Belief in the immediacy of

TABLE 5.1
Classification of factors causing behavior

Behavioral objectives

Within three days of the initial manifestation of sore throat, 80 percent of the children in Hobbit's Preschool Program will have a throat culture done based on a swab taken by a parent.

The target group for the learning objectives will be the parents of the preschoolers and the parents' employers, relatives, and physicians.

Predisposing factors

Positive	Negative
Attitudes, beliefs, and values: Mothers value child's health; mothers have been willing to use health services regularly. Knowledge: Mothers can read thermometers and determine temperatures; children are old enough to report sore throats.	Attitudes, beliefs, and values: Sore throats are not important; mothers feel that sore throats are temporary; mothers feel that sore throats do not have serious consequences and that there is no relationship between strep throat and sequelae.

Reinforcing factors

Positive	Negative
Teachers can identify ill children; teachers relate well to parents; clinical doctor has set up positive interaction with group; teachers and medical personnel will encourage and support parents in taking throat swabs.	Mother's employers not generous about time off for child's illness; grandmothers (baby-sitters) consider sore throats inconsequential and temporary.

Enabling factors

Positive	Negative
Mothers have thermometers in homes; clinic is close by; insurance reduces cost of follow-up visit. Throat swab kit for home use is available; clinic will provide culture and analysis in three days; skill in swabbing is easily learned.	Cost of Rx penicillin regimen; teachers can not take child to doctor; parent has to stay home with child or arrange for sitter because there is no preschool isolation room.

---

the risk and its implications will have to be developed before attention is given to ways to reduce the risk. A family planning service must have its facility in operation and services available before it creates a demand for the services. The enabling factors that provide the services will have to come first. Reinforcement factors can not come into play until behaviors have been evidenced. Predisposing factors would be translated into interventions first.

Some enabling factors may have to be developed over a long period by means of community organization efforts, legislative pressure, and reallocation of resources. When this is the case, the initial concerns of the basic target group may have to be postponed for months.

Some factors may be difficult to work with because of agency policies or mandates. An agency may be restricted to activities related to one set of factors. A hospital may not have the personnel to contact families at home and have to depend on another agency to undertake the task. A school system may be controlled by a board of education ruling that family planning is to be taught only within the context of classes on marriage and the family and that discussion and provision of contraception is not a school responsibility.

Work on several factors can and should proceed simultaneously, however. Cooperation with the appropriate agency to establish a rehabilitation service for alcoholics, for example, can coincide with the mounting of a general information campaign throughout the community on the costs of alcoholism and the efficacy of treatment. By the time the service is operational, the climate is set for specific information about the type and availability of services.

Establishing Priorities Within Categories

Within the three categories of behavioral causes factors can be selected for intervention using the same criteria as were used on the selection of the initial behaviors: importance and changeability.

Importance can be estimated by judging prevalence, immediacy, and necessity according to logic, experience, and available data and theory.

Importance   How widespread or frequent is the factor? If the factor identified is very widespread or occurs often, it should qualify for priority consideration. For example, if 80 percent of the students in a school system believe that smoking is harmless, then dealing with that belief in an antismoking campaign will have a much higher priority than it will if it is shared by only 10 percent of the students.

How compelling or urgent is the factor? Knowing the symptoms of heart attack and what is needed to save a victim's life is one example of knowledge that has immediate consequences for people at high risk of heart attack. Another type of immediacy has to do with how close the connection is between the factor and the group at risk. A certain group of adults believes there to be no connection between strep throat and rheumatic heart disease. Changing that belief is a high priority if the adults holding that belief are the parents of young children who are part of a prevention program. It is not a high priority if the adults are the parents of graduating seniors.

If an outcome cannot be achieved without a certain factor, that factor deserves priority. Knowledge can often be considered necessary (though insufficient) to bring about an action. It is difficult to envision a person's committing himself or herself to a patient role without certain seeds of knowledge, however minimal. Certain beliefs can also be considered necessary. A person who is supposed to present himself or herself for a medical service must have some belief (no matter how faint) that the health professional can help alleviate the problem.[23]

Changeability   Evidence of the changeability of a factor can be gained from looking at the results of previous programs. Assessments of changeability can also be made using techniques set forth in the literature. Rokeach, for example, posits a hierarchy in which beliefs are easier to change than attitudes and attitudes are easier to change than values.[24]

Other planners analyze changeability and priority of factors according to a theory on stages in adoption and diffusion of innovations. This theory is based on work in communications and extensive experience in agriculture, education, family planning, and public health.[25] Behavior change is analyzed over time, and the stages by which behavior is adopted are observed at the individual level and at the social level. Individuals pass through stages labeled "awareness," "interest," "trial," "decision," and "adoption" or, in another version, "knowledge," "persuasion," "decision," and "adoption." When these stages are charted in a population or social system, they follow a pattern of prevalence or cumulative diffusion that looks like a series of increasingly flattened S-shaped curves (fig. 5.2).

In figure 5.2 the five stages of adoption and the four groups of adopters identify points in time when different communication methods and channels are more or less effective. This allows the health educator to match the most appropriate educational strategy with the stage of the program. For example, mass media are most efficient with innovators and early adopters, but outreach methods such as home visits are necessary with late adopters. Depending on the percentage of the population who have already adopted the health behavior at a given point in time, the relative changeability of the behavior in the remaining population is defined by this theory of diffusion.

Observability also influences changeability. If the factor is observable and can be demonstrated, a climate for others is set and their efforts reinforced. As an example, consider the growing emphasis on nonsmoking in group meetings. Mass communications can often be utilized to set up reinfor-

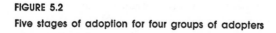

FIGURE 5.2

Five stages of adoption for four groups of adopters

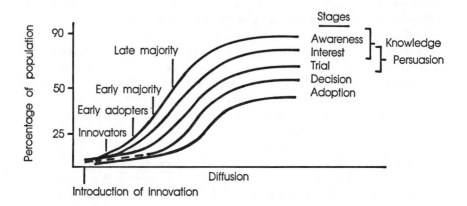

cing climates that support and promote certain behaviors. The function of media in such instances is not to "motivate" but to reinforce.

KEYING LEARNING OBJECTIVES TO THE DIFFUSION PROCESS

Writing learning objectives is similar to writing behavioral objectives, as presented in chapter 4. Such techniques as attitudinal change questionnaires, knowledge quizzes, or, in the case of skills, demonstrations are often used to determine whether the learning objectives have been met.

An example of how learning objectives relate to behavioral objectives is shown in table 5.2. Predisposing and enabling factors analyzed in table 5.1 have been restated in terms of learning objectives for parents. Note the variations in the "how much" in these examples. It is usually possible to create a high level of knowledge; often, over 90 percent of a given population can be made aware of a given fact. Of those who are made aware, a smaller percentage will believe the fact is relevant, important, or useful. Of those who hold these beliefs, not all will develop the requisite skill to carry out the recommended actions. Hence, if 60 percent of the population is expected to adopt the behavior, it is necessary to develop skills in 70 percent, to establish health beliefs in 80 percent, and to create knowledge of the problem or recommendation in 90 percent or more.

This phenomenon accompanies the diffusion of any health practice. Figure 5.3 shows percentages of people over time who are aware that ciga-

TABLE 5.2

Examples of learning objectives based on predisposing and enabling factors analyzed in table 5.1

Problem: Teaching parents to swab sore throats and submit swabs for throat cultures.

1. Knowledge:　By the end of the program period, 90 percent of the parents
   - *a)*　will identify sore throat and fever as potential strep throat.
   - *b)*　will identify throat swabs as necessary to determine whether strep accompanies sore throat.
   - *c)*　can state the cure for strep throat and state that prescriptions are available at the clinic.

2. Beliefs:　　By the end of the program, 80 percent of the parents
   - *a)*　will believe that the consequences of strep throat can be serious.
   - *b)*　will believe that a cure is available.
   - *c)*　will believe that they can take action leading to identification and treatment of strep throat.
   - *d)*　will believe that this series of steps will reduce the potential for further illness.

3. Skills:　　By the end of the program period, 70 percent of the parents
   - *a)*　will be able to swab a child's throat.
   - *b)*　will be able to return swab to clinic laboratory.

---

rette smoking is harmful, who are interested in doing something about it, and who stop smoking. By 1970 between 80 and 90 percent of the target group has become aware of the dangers of smoking; somewhat fewer than 50 percent have been able to adopt the behaviors necessary to end the habit. It is clear at this point that further efforts should be made to increase the number of people willing to try quitting and to help those who want to be successful. Is is also clear that little can be gained by continuing a program whose only emphasis is increasing awareness. This kind of historical analysis can be helpful in establishing an appropriate emphasis for a health program.

One may also observe in figure 5.3 that the diffusion curves for awareness, interest, and adoption of smoking-cessation knowledge, persuasion, and behavior are similar at corresponding stages to the diffusion curves in figure 5.2. If figure 5.3 were extended over a longer period of time, it would show increased rates of adoption of smoking-cessation behavior.

FIGURE 5.3

Adoption curve for smoking cessation—percentages aware, interested, and of former smokers, by age group: United States, 1964, 1966, 1970

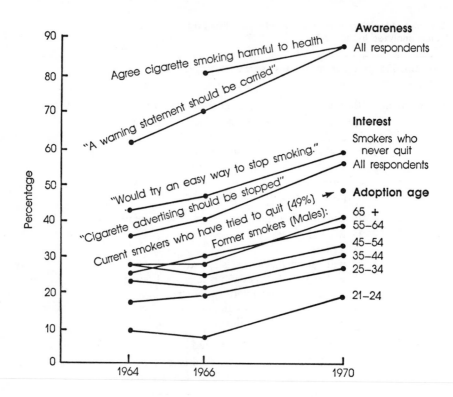

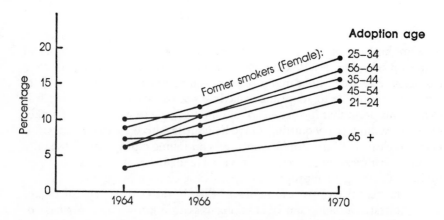

SOURCE: L. W. Green, "Diffusion and Adoption of Innovations Related to Cardiovascular Risk Behavior in the Public," in **Applying Behavioral Science to Cardiovascular Risk,** A. J. Enelow and J. B. Henderson, eds. (New York: American Heart Association, 1975).

SUMMARY

In this chapter we examine the causes of health behavior, calling this phase of PRECEDE the educational diagnosis because we identify those factors on which health education can have a direct and immediate influence. After identifying the factors, we suggest ways that they can be critically assessed as to their relative importance and their relative changeability. Use of these two criteria makes it possible to rank the various causes of health behavior in order of priority and to focus the health education program where it will do the most good in facilitating voluntary adaptations of behavior conducive to health.

EXERCISES

1. For one of the high-priority behaviors you selected in the previous chapter, make an inventory of all the predisposing, enabling, and reinforcing factors you can identify.

2. Rate each factor believed to cause the health behavior according to each of two criteria: importance and changeability. Give each factor a rating of low, medium, or high on each criterion.

3. Write learning objectives for the three highest-priority determinants of the health behavior, one objective for a predisposing factor, one for an enabling factor, and one for a reinforcing factor.

6

Selection of Educational Strategies

ONCE THE BEHAVIORAL DIAGNOSIS has been completed and the health behavior analyzed in terms of its predisposing, reinforcing, and enabling factors, the health educator is ready to plan the health education strategy most suitable for his or her program, with its unique configuration of factors relating to the target group and the health problem. The term *health education strategy* is broadly defined in this chapter to include a combination of methods, approaches, and techniques that may be used to affect the predisposing, reinforcing, and enabling factors which directly or indirectly influence behaviors. Health educators have a broad range of educational means at their disposal, including lectures, group discussions, role playing, mass media,

This chapter is based on "Methods and Strategies in Health Education: A Review of the Literature," a manuscript prepared by Edward E. Bartlett.

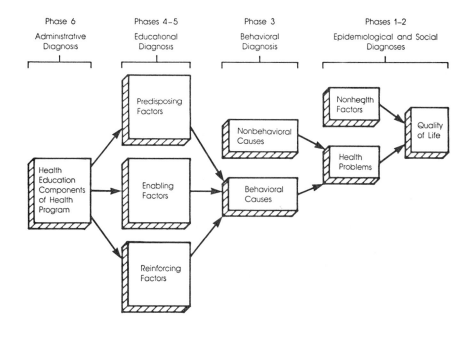

Phase 6	Phases 4–5	Phase 3	Phases 1–2
Administrative Diagnosis	Educational Diagnosis	Behavioral Diagnosis	Epidemiological and Social Diagnoses

and community organizing. In planning an effective program, they must select the best possible combination of educational approaches.

REVIEW OF HEALTH EDUCATION STRATEGIES

It is an educational axiom that a variety of educational methods should be used in trying to achieve an educational end; indeed, we have incorporated this principle into our definition of health education in chapter 1. Nonetheless, many health educators have been caught in a technology trap, committing what we have called the fallacy of the inherently superior method. They continue to use one particular educational approach simply because it has worked well in previous situations or because they are familiar with it. Thus, some health educators consistently favor the lecture method; others rely on group discussion, values clarification, or audiovisual methods of teaching. Some tend to equate health education with a mass media campaign. No one of these methods need be restricted to a particular health education setting. Each can be adapted in a number of ways to a number of situations.

A substantial amount of research has been done on the relative usefulness of different educational methods; health educators in school settings have made the greatest contribution in this area. Research design has generally been based on nonrandomized, matched groups, and outcomes have been measured in terms of knowledge, attitudes, behaviors, and medical improvements (in order of decreasing frequency).

This chapter, in bringing up to date earlier reviews of the literature relating to general communication methods and materials, patient education, and school health education,[1] aims at making explicit the criteria that health educators use in their selection of educational methods. Reviewing the relevant research from the fields of psychology, pedagogy, communications, and community organizing on each health education method will enable the planner to plan his or her programs with a degree of objectivity not otherwise possible.

The educational strategies we describe fall into three broad categories: (1) "communication" methods including lecture-discussion, individual counseling or instruction, the four media techniques of mass media, audiovisual aids, educational television, and programmed learning; (2) training methods including skills development, simulations and games, inquiry learning, small-group discussion, modeling, and behavior modification; (3) and organizational methods including community development, social action, social planning, and organizational development.

Our classification is somewhat arbitrary. Programmed learning, for example, has elements common to individual instruction and audiovisual aids; games often include small-group discussion. Values clarification is not included as a separate educational strategy. (It is approached predominantly by means of small-group discussions and role playing.) Strictly speaking, the organizational methods (community development, social action, social planning, and organizational development) are not of the same scope as the others, each of them encompassing a variety of tactics such as small-group discussions, boycotts, strikes, demonstrations, and areawide health planning. Nonetheless, for purposes of this chapter, the outline is useful.

It is tempting to try to connect each strategy to one class of factors, whether predisposing, reinforcing, or enabling, but it can't be done. There is too much overlap. A strategy can influence two and often three classes of factors. For example, it may at first appear that community-organizing strategies influence only the enabling factors. Further reflection reveals, however, that the participation inherent in the community-development approach is also relevant to the predisposing and reinforcing factors. Generally, the predisposing and enabling factors are influenced by: lecture discussion; individual instruction; mass media; audiovisual aids; programmed learning; educational television; skills development; simulations and games; inquiry learning; small-group discussion; modeling; and behavior modification. Community development, social action, social planning, and organizational development relate primarily to the enabling factors.

No one questions the importance of selecting appropriate educational methods, but one must not lose sight of the fact that the caring teacher is probably more influential in promoting learning than any method. Educational methods are simply the means by which the inspired and committed teacher works to promote the growth and development of the learner. Health education is more than the mechanical selection of educational strategies or the dutiful dissemination of information; its effectiveness depends on the educator's genuine concern for and rapport with the pupil. Indeed, reviews of scores of educational research studies in which one teaching method failed to show a clear-cut advantage over another in improving knowledge have concluded that a "program of instruction may turn out to be a mere incidental feature in the educational process"[2] and that any apparent advantage of new methods can be attributed to their novelty.

Lecture

The lecture is one of the world's oldest formal teaching methods. It is perhaps one of the easiest to use but one of the most difficult to master. The lecture imparts information, influences opinion, stimulates thought, and develops critical thinking through reliance on a verbal message.[3] Learners are usually passive; they generally do not share their knowledge with the teacher or other students. The lecture method is frequently used in conjunction with a question-and-answer period. Its effectiveness is greatly enhanced when students are allowed to clarify their understanding. The common term *lecture-discussion* refers to a combination of information dissemination and questions and answers.

Virtually every experimental study has confirmed the efficacy of the lecture in conveying factual information. What has not been demonstrated, however, is the superiority of the conventional lecture method over discussion groups, educational television, films, or teaching machines. Indeed, several reviews indicate that none of these methods is any more efficacious than any other in the general dissemination of health information.[4] Television, programmed learning, and films were more favorably reviewed than other techniques during the 1950s when they were relatively new.[5]

One study found no significant differences in health knowledge, attitudes, and practices of 900 college freshmen who had been in health education classes with small discussion groups, lecture-discussion groups, or large formal lectures.[6] Other studies indicate that the lecture approach is less effective than group discussion and other educational methods when the educational diagnosis indicates the need for attitudinal change or the development of problem-solving and values-clarification skills. In addition, the cumulative evidence supports the generalization that instructional effectiveness and learner interest are enhanced when a variety of learning methods is employed.[7]

The lecture (and its educational relative, individual instruction) is probably the technique used most by health educators and other health personnel, particularly in school and clinical settings. Its popularity appears to be based on its relative simplicity, adaptability, economy, and practicality. Nonetheless, the lecture method is probably overused, particularly in light of recent improvements in group discussion, programmed learning, and audiovisual techniques, for example. The challenge to health education specialists is to train and provide consultation to nurses, dietitians, pharmacists, dentists, and physicians in the effective use of all educational methods, including the lecture-discussion method.

Individual Instruction

Individual instruction, often referred to as *counseling* in patient settings and commonly used in community health education during home visits, is instruction on a one-to-one basis. The most personalized of all teaching methods, it can be used when the range of individual differences within the target group is great. Individual instruction is inefficient from the point of view of the provider but efficient for the learner.[8]

In school settings, individual instruction has received increased attention from educators dissatisfied with the mass education approach aimed at reaching the "average" learner, thus alienating the slow learner and boring the bright learner. Educators advocate using a diagnosis of a learner's needs as a basis for individualizing an instructional program.

In patient settings, individual counseling by the physician, nurse, or other health professional is the oldest and, according to a recent survey by the American Hospital Association, by far the most common method of health education.[9] Individual instruction also appears to be the predominant method used in home visits. One relatively recent variation on the individual-instruction method is the development of telephone educational programs in which a caller can request to hear recorded tapes of information about cancer or other health problems.[10]

Mass Media

Health educators use four media techniques: mass media, audiovisual aids, educational television, and programmed learning. The media strategies differ from the other approaches we are discussing in that they are not based on face-to-face communications; instead, messages are conveyed through television, radio, charts, posters, manuals, or teaching machines.

Mass media are the channels of communication through which large numbers of people are addressed. Frequently the target group makes little or no effort to receive a message. Common electronic media are radio and television; common print media are magazines, newspapers, and billboards. Mass media are differentiated from the three other media approaches by the relatively large number of people reached, by the fact that a message is a self-contained unit, and by the requirement that a message be relatively simple. They are considered to be relatively *ineffective* means of communication because messages can not be differentiated for specific target groups; but they are considered to be very *efficient* educationally because of the low unit costs achieved by their economy of scale.

Some have advocated that the mass media be used unabashedly to persuade people to adopt salubrious behaviors and that the techniques used by commercial firms to market their products be adopted.[11] If the public can be persuaded to buy particular brands of cigarettes, cars, or mouth washes, why can't that same public be convinced to seek immunizations, have Pap smears done annually, and quit smoking? The reasoning implied by this question fails to appreciate several intrinsic differences between marketing products for consumption and marketing healthy life-styles.

1. The health practices advocated by health educators often are inherently unrewarding, painful, or a nuisance.
2. While corporations simply try to get consumers of competing brands to switch to their own product and to increase the consumption of that product, health educators must often attempt to alter life-styles incorporating noxious habits pursued for years.
3. A corporate advertising campaign is considered successful if 2 or 3 percent of the target audience switches brands, but a public health campaign to control diseases must achieve behavioral change in a majority of the population.
4. Compared to corporate advertising budgets, budgets for health education programs are minuscule.

5. The ethics of promoting health education using the "hidden per-
suaders" techniques of Madison Avenue are an issue for some.

In practice many health education programs do not remotely resemble
Madison Avenue efforts: They are often preachy, boring, unimaginative,
and lacking in artistic appeal. A middle course would be a partial corrective:
Health educators should become more aggressive in adopting some of the
techniques used by marketers and media specialists at the same time they keep
in mind the difficulties inherent in selling their particular "product."

In a classic article "The Role of Mass Media in Public Health," Griffiths
and Knutson summarized three effects of the mass media:

1. increase knowledge
2. reinforce previously held attitudes (but not change contrary
attitudes)
3. cause behavioral change, provided that a psychological predisposition to such an action already exists.[12]

Scores of empirical studies examining the relationship between communications and the diffusion of innovations suggest that the mass media are
most effective in influencing adoption of behavior during the early stages of
the diffusion process.[13] Recent research on the relationship between televised
violence and aggressive behavior suggests that modeling may account for
part of the effect of mass media in facilitating behavioral change.[14] Today's
youth may be exposed to a wide variety of models of attractive behavior that
is different from the behavior of their parents, relatives, and teachers in contrast to children from pre-television days.

The complex problem of which mass media to use for a given program
has occupied the attention of marketers and advertisers for years. Engel,
Wales, and Warshaw have provided a very useful review of the advantages
and disadvantages of each of the major media: television, radio, newspapers,
magazines, outdoor advertising, transit advertising, and direct mailings.[15]

Television is the most "mass" of the mass media, being watched daily
by 92 percent of all American households for a 1972 average per television
household of six hours and ten minutes. Of all the media, television is believed to have the most emotional impact because it combines colorful visual
and auditory messages. National network time can be purchased for between
$5,000 and $15,000 (daytime) and for between $50,000 and $75,000 (prime
time) per commercial minute. Those interested in reaching a narrower audience at less cost can buy time for spot announcements ranging from ten to
sixty seconds in length from local network affiliates. Health education
messages can be broadcast at no charge as public service announcements,
generally during nonprime-time hours. Television programs will likely

reach more selected audiences in the future (as more and more people buy television sets).

Radio reaches as broad an audience as television. Of all U.S. households 99 percent have at least one radio set; and 96.6 percent of the population over the age of twelve listens to the radio at least once a week. In contrast to television, radio has become a very selective medium. Programming can be tailored to the interests and tastes of the local audience. The cost per time unit for radio is one of the lowest of all media, and there is some evidence that radio is very effective for conveying simple material to less educated audiences.

Newspapers are for the most part a local medium. They are read daily in 77 percent of all households (even in those where less than $5,000 is earned annually, 67 percent read newspapers daily) and are believed to inspire greater trust than such nonprint media as television or radio. Recent trends indicate that newspapers will become increasingly localized, segmented, and specialized.

That magazines were once a nonselective medium is epitomized by such general-interest publications as *Look, Life,* and *Saturday Evening Post.* Magazines have now become one of the most selective of all media. Many national magazines even offer regional or demographic editions. One survey found that the average magazine is read by 3.6 adults, each of whom spends an average of eighty-three minutes for this purpose. Magazine reading increases with both education and income. The number of special-interest publications will continue to increase, offering health educators better opportunities to reach at-risk populations.

Outdoor advertising is reputed to be the oldest form of mass media; outdoor signs have been found in the ruins of Pompeii, destroyed in 79 A.D. Outdoor advertising is a flexible medium; it can be used to reach a broad, undifferentiated audience or a more specific target group. This medium reaches upper-income adults most effectively.

Transit advertising on buses and subways is less frequently used than outdoor advertising. It is believed that at least 40 million Americans ride transit vehicles every month. Only half are able to recall inside-vehicle advertising. (The figure is basically the same for all media.) Nevertheless, transit advertising is relatively economical, averaging from $.15 to $.20 per *thousand* inside-vehicle exposures.

Direct mail offers great selectivity in reaching the target audience. A 1972 survey conducted by the U.S. Postal Service found that 65 percent of all direct mail is read immediately and another 14 percent set aside for later reading. Direct mail is considered to be one of the most effective media, an advantage that is somewhat offset by its relatively high cost (from $.12 to $.21 per exposure).

To help the health educator select the most appropriate medium or combination of media, the advantages and disadvantages of these media are rated grossly in table 6.1. The health educator should also consider two other mass media: telephone campaigns and door-to-door requests. Such volunteer groups as the Boy Scouts, Girl Scouts, and 4-H may be very helpful in the door-to-door approach.

The issue of media mix can not be discussed in detail in this book; however, it is revealing to note the percentage allocations of all advertising expenditures in 1973: newspapers (30.3 percent), "miscellaneous" (19.7 percent), television (17.9 percent), direct mail (14.7 percent), radio (6.7 percent), magazines (5.3 percent), and outdoor advertising (1.2 percent).

Considering the high rate of acceptance of mass media as an important health education approach, it is surprising that health educators are not more skilled in their use. Most mass media efforts are directed by communications specialists who produce health education announcements and shows in cooperation with a subject-matter expert. Such programs are generally characterized by superior artistic and technical quality. They are sometimes less effective than they should be, however, because the interests of the audiences have not been assessed and the effort has not been coordinated with other efforts in the community.

Audiovisual Aids

Although superficially similar to the mass media, audiovisual aids (also referred to as *audiovisual techniques*) differ on two counts: scope and comprehensiveness.[16] Audiovisual aids typically reach a more limited audience—children in a classroom, patients in a clinic, or workers at a job site. They are intended only to supplement and reinforce other educational methods, such as lectures, group discussion, games, or behavior modification. Some audiovisual aids are audio only (cassette tapes, records); others are visual (textbooks, charts, posters, diagrams, filmstrips, overhead projections, blackboard, manuals, pamphlets); and many are made up of both audio and visual components (movies, slide-tape programs). With sufficient resources (including knowledge), several of the audiovisual techniques can be used together in a multimedia presentation. Audiovisual aids can be selected according to the criteria outlined in table 6.2 on page 107.

Health textbooks have been judged to have (1) reading levels too high for the intended audience; (2) uniform reading levels throughout an academic year; (3) wide uncontrolled variations in reading levels within and between books developed for the same grade; and (4) low "human interest" scores at higher reading levels.[17] Printed materials used in patient education have also been found to have reading levels too high for most patients.[18]

TABLE 6.1
Mass media rated according to selected criteria

Criterion	Medium						
	Newspaper	Television	Radio	Magazines	Outdoor advertising	Transit advertising	Direct mail
Selectivity	Medium	Low	High	High	Low–medium	Low	High
Cost per person exposure	High	Low (public service announcements)–high (ads)	Low	Medium	Medium	Low	High
Socioeconomic groups most reached	Middle; upper	Lower; middle	All classes	Middle; upper	Middle; upper	Lower; middle	All classes
Age range most reached	Middle; old	Children; old; housewives during day	Teen; old	Young; middle adult	Young; middle adult	All ages	All ages
Complexity of message	High	Medium	Low	High	Low	Low	Medium
Effectiveness per person exposed	Medium	Low–medium	Medium	Medium–high	Low–medium	Low	High

According to Cauffman, films are the most widely used audiovisual aid in school settings. Films are also effective in presenting factual information for a wide variety of ages, topics, and teaching conditions, and most so when accompanied by an introductory presentation of salient principles and a concluding summary.[19] It is also plausible to state, by way of extrapolation from research on the effects of mass media,[20] that films are effective in increasing knowledge, in reinforcing existing attitudes, and in facilitating behavioral change when there is a predisposition to action.

But regarding the *superiority* of one audiovisual technique over another, Campeau in her rigorous review of audiovisual aids used in adult education reaches a more sobering conclusion:

> What is most impressive about the formidable body of literature surveyed for this review is that it shows that institutional media are being used extensively, under many diverse conditions, and that enormous amounts of money are being spent for the installation of very expensive equipment. All indications are that decisions as to which audiovisual devices to purchase, install, and use have been based on administrative and organizational requirements and on considerations of costs, availability, and user preference, *not on evidence of instructional effectiveness*—and no wonder. To date, media research in post-school education has not provided decision makers with practical, valid, dependable guidelines for making these choices on the basis of instructional effectiveness.[21]

Once familiar stock-in-trade of community health educators, audiovisual techniques are less used in contemporary health education practice. Nonetheless, a variety of individualized slide viewers are currently being marketed for use in patient education, and a revival of interest in the use of audiovisual aids in clinical settings is under way. Though such techniques have frequently been overused (and misused) in health education programs, their utility can not be disputed. Patients like them; and they are convenient, low in cost, adaptable, and can be quite effective instructionally.

Programmed Learning

The term *programmed learning* refers to learning brought about by means of teaching machines, programmed tests, and computers, which can be programmed to present materials in a carefully organized sequential system.[22] In contrast to audiovisual materials, which usually play a supporting role, a program presents a complete lesson; a teacher is not needed unless there are questions to be answered. Programmed learning allows learners to progress at their own rates. According to anecdotal reports, it appears to be effective in enhancing learners' motivation. Recent interest in the use of programmed learning has been fostered by a movement in favor of individualized learning experiences and by developments in computer technology.

Small teaching machines came into use during the 1950s under the leadership of B. F. Skinner.[23] These teaching machines actively involved students as they worked through a program step by step, progressing from the known to the unknown in a straight-line sequence. A variation of the linear program, called the branching program, was developed by Norman Crowder. The branching program incorporates alternative paths through a course, depending on the correctness of a student's responses. Students who give wrong answers are shown their errors and subsequently returned to the original or alternate frames to retest their learning.[24]

Because of the high start-up costs of teaching machines and their limited flexibility, they have been all but replaced by printed programmed texts. Programmed texts frequently incorporate branching (or "scrambled") pathways and often are complemented by slides, films, pictures, and tape recordings.

The most recent development in programmed learning is computer-aided instruction (CAI), in which a student works at a terminal in direct ("on-line") communication with a computer. So far, CAI has been employed principally in university settings; decreased production and developmental costs in the future may make CAI suitable for wide-scale use.[25]

Programmed learning appears to be most appropriate when the range of individual differences is great enough to indicate the need for individualized learning; when the subject material is relatively unambiguous, straightforward, and repetitive (e.g., multiplication tables, anatomy, and physiology); when the content is of a confidential or embarrassing nature (e.g., venereal disease, urine sample); and when the necessary funds and expertise exist to set up and operate such a program (particularly so in the case of computer-aided instruction).

Programmed learning has not been used very often by health educators in school settings and has been used even less often in community settings. In clinical settings, however, there have been a number of pioneering efforts. Computers have been used to provide information on venereal disease, dietary problems, diabetes, and obtaining clean-catch urine specimens.[26]

Educational Television

Educational television, like programmed learning, can be used to present self-contained instructional programs, but, unlike programmed learning, it is generally used for an entire class. The programs are either locally developed or nationally broadcast. Occasionally educational television is used to show a "trigger tape," the purpose of which is to stimulate class discussion on a controversial topic. Its acceptance by educators in school settings has paralleled the growth of programmed instruction during the past two decades.

Despite claims to the contrary by its proponents, instruction by means of educational television has not been shown to be superior to other educational methods, although it may save classroom time.[27] Schramm, who reviewed 393 studies comparing the effectiveness of television with other forms of instruction, reported that 255 studies found no significant difference, 83 concluded that television was superior, and 55 demonstrated that traditional classrooms approaches were best.[28]

In spite of these findings, it is reasonable to speculate on the possibility that educational television (as well as programmed instruction) has specific educational advantages in aspects of cognition and psychomotor skills that these studies did not attempt to measure. Future research will undoubtedly shed light on this question.

As in the case of programmed learning, educational television has not been used extensively by health educators in school or community settings, although closed-circuit use has been reported for teaching prepartum and postpartum women in a hospital setting.[29]

In view of the unproved superiority of programmed instruction and educational television over other techniques and in view of their cost, these methods should be used only in controlled experimental settings for the purpose of establishing their effectiveness.[30]

A conclusion such as this, reinforced by similar inconclusive findings on the instructional superiority of lectures, small-group discussions, inquiry learning, and audiovisual aids in effecting cognitive outcomes, supports our view that the critical variables in disseminating factual information may not be restricted to the teaching method or the organization of the material, but may include the appropriate timing and targeting of information based on the diagnostic considerations discussed in the preceding chapters.

Skill Development

Skill development (also referred to as *skill building* or *demonstration*) is a performance-oriented educational method that emphasizes the development of specific psychomotor competencies. Parents' teaching their children to brush their teeth correctly, nutrition education classes in which people learn to cook foods to avoid excessive loss of nutrients, prenatal classes in which breathing techniques are demonstrated, child-care courses in which parents learn to take temperatures rectally, family planning classes that provide instruction in diaphragm insertion, self-help programs detailing techniques for breast self-examination, and nurses instructing diabetic patients on insulin injection—all are examples of skill development.

Optimally, the skill development method includes explanations of the need for a procedure and of how it is done; demonstration of the procedure to the whole group; and opportunities for each student to give a complete explanation and demonstration of the procedure to another student or to the whole group of students.

The skill development method has recently been extended to include use to improve communication skills for conflict resolution, values clarification, and group decision making. The method has also been used in school health education programs to teach teenagers how to say no when they are subjected to peer pressure to smoke cigarettes.

The few evaluations that have been done of the skill development approach generally demonstrate that it can produce significant improvements in psychomotor abilities.

Simulations and Games

Simulation is an experiential method in which a model of a real-life situation is used to stimulate and aid learning.[31] Simulations may take the form of games, dramatization, sociodrama, role playing, case studies, and computerized models. Selected aspects of a real situation are incorporated into the simulation, and time and space are compressed. Although role playing has been used as an educational strategy for years, more sophisticated approaches to simulations have been employed only since the 1960s.

Research is limited, but simulations appear to be suitable for use with learners having a wide range of abilities and to be effective in increasing motivation.[32] They also present abundant opportunities for work in values clarification and in developing empathy skills. The greatest potential of simulation learning appears, then, to be within the affective (attitudinal) domain, even though most health education games developed so far have primarily addressed the cognitive domain.

On the whole, however, simulations have not been widely used by health educators. In a recent issue of *Health Education Monographs* devoted to this topic, Sleet and Stadsklev point out that most health education games are unsuitable for classroom use because they are too simple or too complicated because they take too much time. Still, for those who favor experiential learning, simulation is a promising approach. According to Sleet and Stadsklev, the subject areas with the greatest potential for this type of approach are aging, venereal disease, human sexuality, consumer health, health careers, safety education, and health planning.[33]

Inquiry Learning

In the last two decades, under the leadership of Jerome S. Bruner, another experiential education approach has been emphasized. In this approach, called inquiry learning (and, variously, the *discovery approach, problem solving,* and *immersion learning*), students are encouraged to formulate and test their own hypotheses.[34] The emphasis is on independent thinking and on understanding the process by which knowledge is acquired rather than on knowledge itself. Teachers often use the Socratic method and may serve as resources while students execute classroom or community projects. Inquiry learning is the essence of such teaching techniques as field trips and experiments. It fosters student motivation and, generally, development of the cognitive skills of application, analysis, synthesis, and evaluation, surpassing conventional topical approaches in facilitating critical thinking, democratic cooperation, complex problem solving, and values clarification.[35] One study found that students in problem-solving classes scored significantly higher in tests measuring problem-solving skills than their classmates in lecture classes (differences between the two groups in gains of factual information were not significant, however).[36]

The inquiry learning method has been used predominantly in school settings. Nonetheless, in view of its advantages, it could probably be utilized more frequently in community, occupational, and even clinical settings. In one successful application of the method, Roter encouraged and helped patients to ask their doctors the questions that they had wondered about since their previous visits.[37]

Peer-Group Discussion

The scientific study of the use of small groups for educational purposes goes back to the 1930s when Kurt Lewin experimented with the effect of small groups on attitudinal and behavioral changes[38] and when the workshop method of learning and teaching was first being employed.[39] Bond's classical study in 1956 demonstrated the superiority of the discussion-decision method over the lecture method in convincing women to examine their breasts and to receive breast examinations from their physicans, as measured thirteen months after the health education program.[40] Currently, small-group processes are utilized in a broad range of professions and settings for a broad range of purposes, including group psychotherapy, team building, organizational development, community organizing, values clarification, sensitivity training, and wide-scale health promotion and political indoctrination in China.[41]

A number of studies have demonstrated the advantage of group-discussion methods over lectures in developing positive health practices and enhancing long-term motivation among individuals although gains in knowledge are about the same with the two educational strategies.[42] A study by Radke and Caso of 850 junior high school students demonstrated the effectiveness of the discussion-decision method over the lecture approach in improving students' self-reported lunch practices, as measured six and ten weeks after the program.[43]

Modeling

The term *modeling* refers to the human inclination to imitate human behaviors. Modern conceptions of modeling draw on psychoanalytic and role theories of identification and particularly on Bandura's studies of observational learning.[44] Modeling is probably the principal process through which socialization occurs.

Observational learning is not limited to mere mimicry; as shown by studies of language development in chidren, it also results in the development of conceptual rules that allow for adaptation of the learned behavior to novel situations.[45] A person's attraction as a role model increases with his or her perceived power, attractiveness, warmth, and success in gaining rewards.[46]

Although modeling has not been considered traditionally as a teaching method, one can realize its importance by considering the vast influence parents and teachers have on young children. Modeling seems to begin in infancy and continue throughout adult life, although it has the strongest effects early in life. Women appear to be more strongly affected than men, as revealed in sex differences in measures of affiliation and conformity.[47]

Of late, an abundance of studies have focused on the deleterious effects of televised violence on children.[48] It does appear that modeling can be a force for good as well as ill and that it can be decisive in teaching healthy behaviors and establishing good habits, particularly in preschool and early elementary school years. It follows that modeling can play a much greater role than it has in the promotion of healthful practices regarding diet, smoking, use of alcohol, and exercise.[49]

Behavior Modification

Behavior modification is the modification of specific behaviors according to the principles of classical and operant conditioning. In theories of classical conditioning, behaviors are thought to be caused by stimuli (or antecedents). An ashtray, a refrigerator, and a television advertisement are examples of stimuli. In theories of operant conditioning, the frequency of a behavior is thought to be influenced by the consequences of that behavior. The consequences can be positive (which rewards the behavior), nonexistent (which extinguishes the behavior), or negative (which punishes the behavior). Behavior modification, then, is based on the concepts of stimulus control and management of rewards and punishments, a combination deriving from both sets of theories. Experimental successes with animals have been difficult for the most part to replicate with human beings. Notable exceptions have been with people of low IQ, children, and schizophrenics. Trivial behaviors that do not require thought have also been altered successfully.

Essential aspects of cognitive and behavioral psychology have recently been integrated in a learning approach called cognitive behavior modification.[50] Cognitive behavior modification differs from strict behavior modification insofar as it allows for the intervention of cognitive processes (such as decision making, values clarification, thought control, and imagery and attitude change) between stimulus and response. A variety of therapeutic techniques are used in this approach, including counter conditioning, thought stopping, covert sensitization, covert reinforcement, extinction, and modeling. Although this approach is relatively new, it promises to have greater flexibility and effectiveness than either behavior modification or cognitive therapies used alone.

Some health educators demonstrate an almost Pavlovian aversion to the use of behavior modification techniques. It would be advantageous if, instead, they would evaluate behavior modification on its own merits and judge its worth by its benefits to the target group. Behavior modification has rarely been used in community settings; its use in school settings has been restricted to the treatment of learning and emotional disorders by clinical psychologists. Its use in patient settings has been more widespread. One form of behavior modification—client-contract behavior modification—has great potential for use as a health education strategy. In this form the patient voluntarily enters the program, is fully informed of the methods used, decides on and makes an open commitment to a degree of desired behavior change, and has full freedom to withdraw from the program at any time.

Behavior modification has had encouraging results in the treatment of a broad range of clinical problems, including disorders of the genitourinary, gastrointestinal, cardiovascular, musculoskeletal, nervous, and respiratory systems.[51] Foreyt has recently edited a book describing various behavioral treatments of obesity.[52] In another review, Bass reports the use of behavior modification techniques in the treatment of mental retardation, neuroses, psychoses, anorexia nervosa, childhood autism, chronic pain, depression, hysteria, phobias, poor study habits, stuttering, obesity, alcoholism, and cigarette smoking.[53] Of the last three conditions, behavior modification has been the most successfully and widely used in the treatment of obesity; alcoholism and smoking have been less susceptible to long-term improvement by this means (or any other). It may be easier to get people to lose weight than it is to get them to quit smoking because of social factors. The result of over-eating is highly visible, and being obese is socially unacceptable. The obese patient is constantly subjected to negative social pressures. In contrast, the physical effects of smoking are much less observable.

The effectiveness of cognitive behavior modification is less extensively documented. Mahoney cites numerous studies tending to validate it as a method; but virtually all of them were based on a very small sample size (many are individual case studies) and conducted without control groups.[54]

Behavior modification procedures are for changing frequent and com-plex behaviors (habits) that can not be altered through cognitive control (will power), but they can not be implemented successfully without a trained ther-apist and a highly motivated target group. Supportive social norms and pres-sures may be important, as we have suggested. In the final analysis, behavior modification is an extreme measure and should be regarded as the educational method of last resort, to be used only when less costly, simpler methods such as lectures, group discussions, individual counseling, and appropriate mass media campaigns are ineffective.

Community Development

Community development (also referred to as *locality development*), is a process-oriented method of community organizing that emphasizes the development of skills, abilities, and understanding in an entire community for the purpose of social improvement.[55] Community development is based on the self-help, consensus approach to problem solving, and it works best in areas with rec-oncilable interests and compatible social groups. The community organizer serves primarily as a facilitator in the development of problem-solving skills and as a coordinator of improvement programs.

The community development approach is a commonly used commu-nity organizing method, particularly in rural settings. Health education and community development have traditionally been a part of state cooperative extension service programs, with an emphasis on nutrition education, home-making skills, development and coordination of health services, organization of voluntary prepaid health plans, and overall improvement of the conditions of rural life.[56] A family and self-help education program in Oregon sought, among other goals, to help "communities or individual citizens acquire skills and experience in identifying community health education deficits and devel-oping programs to reduce the deficits."[57] Another rural health education pro-gram, in North Carolina, was successful in passing a bond referendum to ex-pand the county hospital.[58] Community development methods have also been used by health educators in Ethiopia as part of an integrated program directed at improvement of health, nutrition, family planning, and agriculture;[59] in Cuba to improve general public health conditions; in Brazil to improve the nutritional status of children under four years of age, using Paulo Freire's "problem-posing" method of education; in Yugoslavia to improve a village water supply; in an Arab village in Israel to eradicate a scabies epidemic; and in Sri Lanka during a cholera outbreak.[60] Indeed, the recent self-help movement shares many methods and goals with the community development approach.[61]

The evaluation of community organizing programs is more difficult than the assessment of other health education methods and approaches because there frequently are unanticipated results, because the effects of these programs are long term, and because the difficulties in differentiating between program and nonprogram effects on outcomes are virtually insuperable. Accordingly, anecdotal case studies are the most common mode of evaluation.

Social Action

Social action is a mode of community organizing in which a disadvantaged segment of a population organizes to make demands for a redistribution of resources.[62] Social action is quite different from community development. Consensus is not assumed to exist among social classes in the community. Members of the target group are seen as unwitting victims of powerful economic and political interest groups. Further, social action is task oriented, and tactics such as rallies, marches, boycotts, and strikes are commonplace. Social action is the method used by such groups as the Congress of Racial Equality, Students for a Democratic Society, and Saul Alinsky's Chicago Woodlawn Organization in the 1960s.

Health professionals use other community organizing approaches more often than social action, perhaps because social action represents too radical a departure from their philosophies, skills, or mandates.

Social Planning and Organizational Development

Social planning, the third principal community organizing strategy, is the process by which experts solve social problems through rational deliberation and change controlled by experts.[63] Basic to the social planning approach are data-gathering and rational problem-solving techniques and the achievement of goals within an institutional context. Social planning is the method used by city planners, welfare councils, community health planners, policy makers and high-level administrators.

Organizational development, a similar approach to problem solving, is the implementation of planned changes within organizations. Organizational development as an approach has been influenced by the group dynamics methods associated with the National Training Laboratory in Bethel, Maine, which began to be used in business, industrial, and school settings in the 1940s.[64] The main techniques of organizational development are team building, conflict management, technostructural changes, data feedback, and training.[65] Writing specifically for health education, Mico and Ross have suggested that these techniques be used to achieve effective working coalitions between institutions, agencies, and power groups within a community.[66]

Training and consultation have long been recognized as intrinsic to the role of the health educator, and two recent issues of *Health Education Monographs* were devoted to these topics.[67] One issue included an analysis of a program to train the members of consumer advisory groups of six hospitals to improve their decision-making skills as well as their overall knowledge of board functioning.[68] Health education specialists have extensive experience in the training of board members of health systems agencies; one such program oriented more than 380 board and staff members from New York, New Jersey, Puerto Rico, and the Virgin Islands.[69] Another example is a training program directed to team building among health science students in rural Appalachia.[70] Organizational development is typically addressed to enabling factors. In a clinic it may include replacing a block appointment system for patients with a staggered appointment system, centralizing the appointment-making mechanism, assigning nurses and physicians to the clinic on a permanent basis, and developing bilingual appointment cards. Such organizational changes in the metabolic clinic of a New Jersey hospital resulted in an improvement of the clinic's kept appointment rate from 52 percent to 71 percent.[71]

A GUIDE FOR LINKING EDUCATIONAL METHODS TO DIAGNOSTIC CRITERIA

We have reviewed the state of the art in the applications of fifteen educational strategies to health education. Now it is possible to present a guide to how these strategies fit in with the major diagnostic categories.

This guide, for convenience broken down into four separate tables (tables 6.2–6.5) breaks the diagnostic phases into four major classifications of variables: (1) those relating to the health problem; (2) those relating to the desired health behavior; (3) those relating to the target group; and (4) those relating to administrative factors. Information regarding the health problem (table 6.2) is derived from the epidemiological diagnosis (chap. 3), that regarding the characteristics of the target group (tables 6.3 and 6.4) from the behavioral and educational diagnoses (chaps. 4 and 5), and that regarding the administrative factors (table 6.5) from the administrative diagnosis (chap. 7). Pertinent to each phase of PRECEDE are several key variables, or diagnostic "criteria," component variations or categories of a variable, and corresponding optimal educational strategies. The target group variables include characteristics of the behavioral problem (table 6.3) and the predisposing, enabling, and reinforcing factors causing the health behavior (table 6.4). The attitudes of family, employers, peers, and health providers (reinforcing factors) toward the target group deserve special educational efforts, and these influential people are specified as a secondary or indirect target group for the program. In table 6.4, target group variables may relate either to the people whose health is at risk or to the people who can influence the behavior of those people.

Health educators using this guide should keep in mind several important points.

1. The relationships are, to a large degree, hypothetical, being based on experience and extrapolations from research done under widely diverse educational conditions.
2. Those relationships extrapolated from experimental evidence are subject to modification as new research is completed.
3. The research was done predominantly in North America and thus, can not be freely applied in cross-cultural situations.
4. The guide is general; numerous exceptions may be found in individual circumstances. Further, because it is general, many of the details and qualifications mentioned in the preceding reviews of each educational strategy have not been incorporated. When none of the fifteen methods appears to offer a clear-cut advantage in influencing a particular dimension, then "no specific recommendations" is indicated.

Though at the present time the guide is somewhat unwieldy, it is potentially practical for the educator who wants to choose his or her methods rationally. It imposes at least a provisional order on what might appear at times to be a bewildering welter of information. It makes explicit the reasons for using an educational method where such use has often been haphazard or based on implicit reasons that were not understood or documented. *

---

*Making the rationale for selection of methods more explicit makes it possible to test and challenge the validity of the assumptions. Theories represented in these tables can thus be subjected to continuous refinement.

TABLE 6.2

Educational strategies according to characteristics of the health problem

Diagnostic criterion	Prevalent category	Audiovisual aids	Lecture	Individual instruction	Mass media	Programmed learning	Educational television	Skill development	Simulations and games	Inquiry learning	Peer-group discussion	Modeling	Behavior modification	Community development	Social action	Social planning and organizational change	No recommendations
Etiology of problem	Primarily environmental, economic													X	X	X	
	Primarily medical or behavioral	X	X	X	X	X	X	X	X	X	X	X	X				
Stage of intervention	Primary prevention	X	X	X	X	X		X			X	X					
	Secondary prevention (reduction in delay in seeking health care)	X		X							X	X					
	Treatment and rehabilitation	X	X			X	X				X		X				
	Post-treatment follow-up			X*	X												
Degree of scientific and social consensus on etiology and priority problem	Low										X	X					
	High		X		X	X	X										
Confidential nature of the illness or problem	Confidential	X		X													
	Nonconfidential																X

*Home visits

TABLE 6.3

Educational strategies according to characteristics of the health behavior

Diagnostic criterion	Prevalent category	Recommended educational strategies															
		Audiovisual aids	Lecture	Individual instruction	Mass media	Programmed learning	Educational television	Skill development	Simulations and games	Inquiry learning	Peer-group discussion	Modeling	Behavior modification	Community development	Social action	Social planning and organizational change	No recommendations
Educational outcome desired	Cognitive: knowledge comprehension	X	X	X	X	X	X		X	X	X						
	Cognitive: application, analysis, synthesis and evaluation								X	X	X						
	Affective								X	X	X						
	Psychomotor							X				X	X				
Complexity of the health information	Simple				X	X	X										
	Complex								X	X	X						
Complexity of the health behavior	Simple	X			X												
	Complex			X									X				
Duration of the health behavior	Short term	X	X		X												
	Long term							X			X	X	X	X	X	X	
Frequency of the health behavior	Infrequent			X	X												
	Frequent							X			X	X	X				
Extent of the health behavior	Rare																X
	Widespread							X						X			
Additive vs. substitutive nature of health behavior	Additive			X								X					
	Substitutive							X			X			X			
Promptness vs. delay of the health behavior	No delay				X												
	Delay																X

TABLE 6.4

Educational strategies according to factors predisposing, enabling, and reinforcing the behavior

Diagnostic criterion	Prevalent category	Audiovisual aids	Lecture	Individual instruction	Mass media	Programmed learning	Educational television	Skill development	Simulations and games	Inquiry learning	Peer-group discussion	Modeling	Behavior modification	Community development	Social action	Social planning and organizational change	No recommendations
Age	Infants and preschool children							X	X	X		X					
	Primary school children	X	X*	X	X			X	X	X	X	X					
	Secondary school children; adolescents	X	X	X	X	X	X		X	X	X	X					
	Adults		X	X						X	X		X				
Educationally disadvantaged	Yes			X		X	X							X	X	X	
	No																X
Social structure	Cohesive, well-integrated													X			
	Noncohesive, poorly integrated			X												X	
Homogeneousness of population	Yes					X											
	No			X													
Beliefs in severity and suscepti-bility to the disease	Weak					X					X						
	Moderate	X	X														
	Strong					X					X						
Socio-economic status	High; inter-mediate				X (print)											X	
	Low				X (electronic)									X	X		

*Lecture-discussion

(continued on next page)

TABLE 6.4 continued

Diagnostic criterion	Prevalent category	Recommended educational strategies															
		Audiovisual aids	Lecture	Individual instruction	Mass media	Programmed learning	Educational television	Skill development	Simulations and games	Inquiry learning	Peer-group discussion	Modeling	Behavior modification	Community development	Social action	Social planning and organizational change	No recommendations
Stage in diffusion process	Innovators and early adopters				X												
	Middle majority		X*											X			
	Late adopters			X†											X		
Motivation	Low		X						X	X	X					X	
	High	X			X	X						X			X		
Social acceptability of desired behavior	Low		X								X						
	High				X												
Individual vs. group orientation of target population or person	Individual (isolated)			X**													
	Group (highly involved)								X	X							
Size of target population	Segment of community													X			
	Total community														X	X	
Stage in adoption process	Awareness; interest		X		X												
	Trial; evaluation; adoption			X							X	X					
Expected degree of adherence to therapeutic regimen	Low		X								X		X	X	X	X	
	High	X	X	X	X												

*Lecture-discussion   †Home visits   **Outreach (home visit, direct mail)

TABLE 6.5

Educational strategies according to administrative considerations

Diagnostic criterion	Prevalent category	Audiovisual aids	Lecture	Individual instruction	Mass media	Programmed learning	Educational television	Skill development	Simulations and games	Inquiry learning	Peer-group discussion	Modeling	Behavior modification	Community development	Social action	Social planning and organizational change	No recommendations
Focus of program: single or multiple health problems or goals	Single health problem															X	
	Noncategorical multiple health problems or goals													X	X		
Time frame of objectives	Short term	X	X	X	X	X	X	X	X		X		X				
	Long term											X		X	X	X	
Program to be evaluated rigorously	No				X				X	X	X			X	X	X	
	Yes	X	X	X		X	X	X			X		X				
Academic background of program directors	Psychology										X	X	X				
	Community organizing and social work													X	X	X	
	Communications	X			X												
	Education	X	X	X		X	X	X	X	X							
	Nursing/ medicine	X	X	X				X									
Support of other community organizations	Yes															X	
	No													X	X		
Health provider's relevant behavior observable by target group	Yes											X					
	No				X												

(continued on next page)

TABLE 6.5 continued

Diagnostic criterion	Prevalent category	Recommended educational strategies															
		Audiovisual aids	Lecture	Individual instruction	Mass media	Programmed learning	Educational television	Skill development	Simulations and games	Inquiry learning	Peer-group discussion	Modeling	Behavior modification	Community development	Social action	Social planning and organizational change	No recommendations
Degree of financial support relative to magnitude of health problem	Minimal	x			x*												
	Great			x	x**	x	x										
Institutional setting of program mature and cohesive	Yes													x	x		
	No															x	
Commitment of local power structure(s) to solving health problem	Little													x			
	Great													x		x	
Interests of community groups and organizations reconcilable	Yes													x		x	
	No														x		

*Press releases, public service announcements, and interviews
**Project-financed television and radio programs

Sometimes, depending on the circumstances, it might be desirable to rate individual criteria quantitatively. The educator reviews the first criterion; he or she then selects the variation of the criterion most closely matching the characteristics of the health problem, the health behavior, the target group, and the administrative/environmental situation and assigns it a numerical value. For example, the coordinator of a kindergarten through twelfth-grade program would select in reviewing the criterion of age the primary and secondary level, giving one point (or more if different values are attached to different criteria) to each strategy suggested. Each criterion is reviewed and rated in the same way. When the review is complete, the points are added. If the criteria have not been differentially weighted, the planner simply makes a list of the strategies most often selected. Finally, he or she, with reference to a few rules of thumb (following) decides on the strategies appropriate to the situation. It is possible that the strategies scoring the highest number of points will not be compatible with the situation. Gross incompatibility could stem from failure to appreciate the hypothetical, general nature of the guide or from a faulty rating scheme. In such a case, the planner must, of course, use his or her best judgment. It should be noted that audiovisual aids are generally not considered in the tables because they are universally used as an adjunct of the other educational methods.

RULES OF THUMB FOR USING THE GUIDE

In the final selection of strategies from among those surfacing in the review of criteria outlined in tables 6.2 through 6.5, it is helpful to keep the following points in mind:

1. Select a *minimum* of three educational strategies for any health education class. For a school health education program, a common combination would be lecture-discussion, small-group discussions or inquiry learning, and audiovisual aids. This rule of thumb is based on the educational axioms that people learn in different ways and that using a variety of teaching approaches increases learner interest. Make sure that all factors—predisposing *and* enabling *and* reinforcing factors—receive attention.
2. In most health education programs, audiovisual aids or other media techniques should be one of the three strategies used. They are effective in reinforcing and strengthening other educational strategies.
3. The longer the health education program (both in terms of hours and number of sessions), the greater the number of educational strategies that should be used.
4. A program is best begun with the simpler, cheaper educational methods such as lecture-discussions, individual instruction, and audiovisual aids that influence the predisposing factors. If these

strategies are unsuccessful, more sophisticated and expensive approaches such as behavior modification, small-group discussions,
and community organizing strategies that affect reinforcing and
enabling factors can be applied.
5. The more complex the causes of the behavioral problem, the greater
the range of strategies that will be required. For example, a program
to advise people in a rural community of the time and place of an im-
munization clinic need consist only of placing a few notices in the local post office, general store, and church. A program to control venereal disease, drug abuse, or teenage pregnancies will require, on
the other hand, massive information-dispensing efforts and community organizing strategies in schools, clinics, work sites, and
other community locations; and these activities must be coordinated
with those growing out of other health, educational, and economic
development programs.
6. Educational strategies that influence predisposing factors only will
generally have only short-term effects; strategies that influence
reinforcing factors will have intermediate effects. Programs that are
designed to influence predisposing, reinforcing, *and* enabling factors
will have the greatest payoffs in long-term behavioral changes.
Note, however, that strategies selected to influence predisposing
factors will generally be simpler and less expensive than those intended to influence reinforcing, and, particularly, enabling factors.

SUMMARY

After completing the diagnostic steps described in chapters 2–5, the information compiled should be used to select the most appropriate educational
methods and strategies. This chapter reviews the state of the art in educational methodologies and the evidence concerning their relative effectiveness
under varied circumstances; it also presents guidelines to the appropriate selection, mixing, and sequencing of methodologies.

It is not our intent in this chapter that students or practitioners memo-
rize long lists of methods and their associated conditions of success. Rather, it
is our purpose to extend the logic of educational diagnosis to the planning of
the educational treatment and to present that logic in a way that will make the
selection of educational methods a natural extension of the previous diagnostic steps.

Even if use of the crude guidelines we offer does not result in the identification of the methods that will have the greatest success in a given situation,

it will ensure that the assumptions behind a selection of methods are made explicit. Given this, the failures and successes of health education can be examined more critically and programs improved more readily.

EXERCISES

1. For the population and health problem you have analyzed, identify three educational methods that would appear to be most appropriate.

2. Justify your selection on the basis of the criteria of tables 6.1–6.5.

3. If you do not have at least one method each directed at predisposing, enabling, and reinforcing factors, add one or more methods to your selection to be sure that all three major determinants of the priority health behavior are addressed by your program.

4. Suggest and justify a sequence for the implementation of your selected educational strategies.

7

Administrative Diagnosis: Assessing Organizational Problems

ONE MORE PHASE of the PRECEDE framework remains to be considered before program implementation: the administrative diagnosis. Administrative considerations include budgeting and analysis of the factors that will determine the ease with which a program is introduced into a system. Although the administrative diagnosis is presented near the end of the planning process, it is important to keep the procedures clearly in mind beginning with the earliest assessment of problems. The extent of the problems analyzed in the early phases of PRECEDE will significantly affect the way resources will be allocated.

In one sense, the material in this chapter is simply a recasting into an administrative context of material already presented. The advice on the selection of methods as well as all the steps in the social, epidemiological, beha-

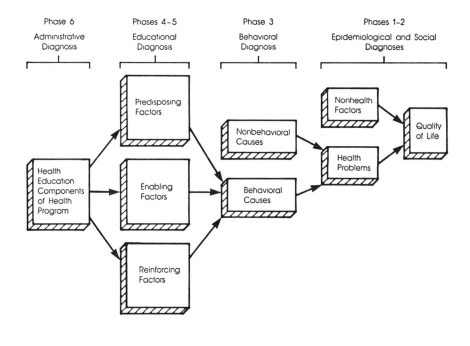

Phase 6
Administrative
Diagnosis

Phases 4–5
Educational
Diagnosis

Phase 3
Behavioral
Diagnosis

Phases 1–2
Epidemiological and Social
Diagnoses

Predisposing
Factors

Enabling
Factors

Reinforcing
Factors

Health
Education
Components
of Health
Program

Nonbehavioral
Causes

Behavioral
Causes

Nonhealth
Factors

Health
Problems

Quality
of Life

vioral, and educational diagnoses have been given at least implicitly in the service of efficient and effective allocation of resources. At the same time that the various factors involved in planning a health education program have been considered in and of themselves, they have been considered generally in terms of their contribution to program success. But no program can be completely successful without an honest appraisal of organizational limitations. Once these are determined, the planner can take steps to overcome them or to compensate for them through relationships with other organizations in the community. The administrative diagnosis, then, analyzes factors that will determine problems or opportunities in the administration of the program, just as the educational diagnosis analyzed factors determining behavioral problems.

RESOURCE ALLOCATION

Budgetary decisions are made according to how best to maximize the use of scarce resources. Decision makers must always, implicitly or explicitly, measure the cost of a program (what must be given up?) against its effects (what will be accomplished?). As part of this process, decisions are also made regarding the merit of the effects and how best to achieve the effects. Essentially, budgetary decisions, calling for adding, cutting back, or modifying existing programs, set organizational priorities.

Budgeting is one way of estimating the resources required to accomplish the objectives of a program. Ideally, a budget permits there to be sufficient resources on hand to meet desired goals, neither too little (necessitating program curtailment) nor too much (resulting in a surplus of funds that could have been allocated elsewhere). The planner, at this point, specifies how the program will be structured, the number of people needed to carry it out, and the necessary equipment and materials. Estimates are based on these specifications.

In health education the major consideration for the budget is personnel. How much effort and time will be required? What kinds of skills and capabilities are needed? What, specifically, are the tasks? Detailed answers to these questions will yield a basic outline of personnel requirements.

In estimating the time required for the health program, the planner must include an estimate of time needed for ongoing organizational maintenance. Maintenance time is, for example, time spent in staff meetings, on training and development of staff members, and in meeting reporting requirements. Each of these activities reduces the time available for program implementation and increases personnel requirements.

Decisions on the levels of skill and experience that will be needed to carry out program tasks may have to be made in consultation with a personnel department, particularly if job descriptions and salary schedules have already been established, as is true in many organizations. Whether people already employed can be reassigned, whether new employees with requisite skills can be recruited, and which of these require training—all are matters to be explored. Findings can affect the length of the lead time for implementation.

Program timing is an important aspect of planning the budget. Selecting and training staff members and getting organized can sometimes take as long as six months. Costs for personnel and materials may thus be less during the first budget period than in subsequent periods, when the full impact of implementation is reflected. A similar situation can obtain when a program is winding down. A useful tool for plotting the time requirements of a program is PERT (Program Evaluation and Review Technique),[1] a way to analyze events in terms of critical paths.

FIGURE 7.1

The allocation of time following the logic of PERT

First three months:
Administrative
activities
required to
start services

Second three months:
Service
activities
required to
reach objectives

Third three months:
Intermediate
objectives
required to
reach target

Final three months:
One-year target

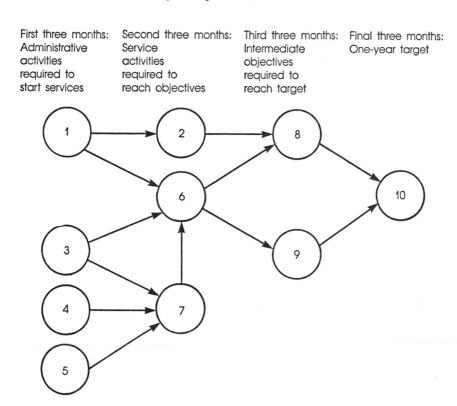

Figure 7.1 shows an example of a PERT diagram. First, the aim of the program after a certain period of time, in this case, one year, is specified (10); then the tasks that will achieve that end are specified (8 and 9); then the steps, procedures, or activities necessary to 8 and 9 are identified (2 and 6); and so forth. The procedure is continued until one arrives at the present or the beginning of the fiscal year. The chief utility of the PERT form of charting is that it helps planners set priorities and establish rough timetables for activities and makes it possible to anticipate fluctuations in resource needs.

The specifics of budgeting, of course, vary according to organization, but the major cost categories, in addition to salaries for personnel and fringe benefits, usually are travel, materials, equipment, and supplies. Quite often, the costs for consultants and specific subcontracts are considered separately,

TABLE 7.1
Sample budget

Personnel

Position	Name	Percentage effort	Salary	Personnel benefits	Total
Director	Dr. James Killer	100	$26,000		
Assistant director	To be named	50	10,000		
Secretary	To be named	50	4,500		
Outreach workers			20,000		
			$60,500	$10,285	$70,785

Consultation
    Fees
        5 days @ $300 $1,500
        2 days @ $400   800
    Travel and per diem
        3 round trips to
        San Francisco   1,500   3,800

Supplies
    Printing and postage   700
    Office supplies,
        books, reprints   350
    Educational materials
        and equipment   2,000   3,050

Services
    Telephone   400
    Photocopying   600
    Data processing   2,500   3,500

Travel
    Local travel   675
    National conferences (2)   1,100   1,775

                                  Total: Direct costs   82,910

Indirect costs (17 percent of total direct costs)   13,894

                                  TOTAL COSTS   **$96,804**

as are overhead administrative costs. Table 7.1 shows a sample budget format.

A budget is always an estimate, subject to negotiation and revision as it is worked out. Accurate budgeting is an art as well as a skill, and practice brings improvement. Inexperienced planners can increase the reliability of their efforts by talking with a wide variety of people, including those who have established similar programs in the past.

Should a budget be based on what it appears the traffic will bear the first year, or should it be complete, covering all expenditures necessary to accomplishing the total program? Working out an ideal budget in the beginning is a valuable exercise. It gives the planner a clear idea of what the program should be like as a whole and allows for systematic planning for what is desired. In contrast, limited planning may result in missed opportunities to use available resources or to achieve potential benefits or in haphazard additions to a program. Further, it may hinder the search for new resources or innovative ways to fill resource requirements.

THE ADMINISTRATIVE DIAGNOSIS

"Producing" a health program can be likened to producing a successful stage play. Mounting a stage production requires, in addition to a polished script and the right combination of talented performers, months of tedious preparation and repeated rehearsals. Lighting, temperature control, amplification mix, props, music, advertising, ticket sales, and countless other elements must be attended to and all these efforts coordinated and completed if a program is to have a fair chance of succeeding. Nothing is left to the last moment, and as little as possible is left to chance. Careful planning and attention to seemingly insignificant details are a hallmark of a good production company. Its internal workings, many of them totally in the background, are critical to the success of its public offerings. So too with health education programs. Planners must pay careful attention to internal organizational details if a program is to be successful.

If health education programs operated autonomously, there would be little demand for intensive administrative planning and coordination. But they are rarely conducted in isolation from other health-related activities. Typically, educational interventions complement and support other efforts to resolve health problems. It is not uncommon for a number of health professionals to assist in program development and delivery. The educational component of a health-enhancing effort may be delivered over an extended period or at intervals rather than only at one time. Formal, planned health education is still relatively unusual. Although numerous instances of health instruction can be identified, there are relatively few systematic, coordinated educational programs with objectives spelled out and evaluation components built in. Many health professionals and administrators have not worked specifically with health education specialists and, in some cases, have never formally included health education as a significant feature of their overall health programs.

That such situations are perfect breeding grounds for overlapping and misdirected efforts, squandered resources, and generalized confusion underscores the utility of a thorough analysis of the organizational context in which the health education will take place. Administrative diagnosis will help the health professional to identify likely impediments as well as facilitators and suggest ways to minimize one and maximize the other.

As we have indicated, educational programs function by means of an extraordinarily wide range of organizational structures. They may be small, independent, community based projects concerned with one specific health issue, or they may be large, complex educational units within large organizations. This discussion will center on a model of a health education program that is part of a larger health project. (*Health education program*, as we are using the term here, refers to a planned educational endeavor, complete with objectives and evaluation.) Not surprisingly, the position of the educational component in the organization, the position of the health professional in charge of the program, and the relationship of the total health project to the overarching agency or organization of which it is a part are important factors influencing the administrative diagnosis.

As one begins an administrative analysis, it is well to remember, as pointed out in the literature on planned change and organization development, that new programs can be viewed as innovations within a system.[2] The introduction of a new element into a system will require adjustments throughout the system. Sometimes the adjustments will have positive effects, sometimes, negative. In wanting to subdue the negative, the conscientious educator will be mindful of the need to become familiar with the agency and community of which his or her project is a part. He or she should allow plenty of time for informal visits in the agency, taking the opportunity to collect organizational charts, assess staff interests and concerns, list the communication channels observed, and construct (mentally) sociograms of the relationships within the agency. At the same time, it is useful to discuss the planned educational program with various staff members and assess how they might contribute to a team effort. The purpose of these activities is to allow the educator to tailor the program as closely as possible to existing efforts and to avoid the difficulties inherent in working at cross purposes.

THREE LEVELS OF DIAGNOSIS

Planners will want to analyze administrative and organizational factors from three distinct perspectives: within the program; within the organization; and between organizations.

Within-Program Analysis

The initial level of administrative diagnosis, the within-program analysis, deals with factors pertaining to the health education program itself, whether it stands alone or is part of a larger health project (fig. 7.2). The factors to be considered are four: (1) the size and complexity of the health education program and of the health project; (2) physical and organizational placement of the health education program; (3) staffing; and (4) space, funding, and general support systems.

Small programs requiring few staff members, all of whom have similar backgrounds, are usually relatively easily implemented because they require less day-to-day attention and because they engender less resistance within the sponsoring organization. In contrast, programs that have a large number of personnel, many different disciplines, several agencies, and a large target population require significant amounts of administrative attention to ensure that personnel are familiar both with the program and with what is expected of them. Lead time for implementation of such a program is longer than usual, owing to the need for complex planning and for thorough interpretation of the program to the organization. Care should be taken to keep communication between program staff members and organization staff members open and easy.

FIGURE 7.2
Focuses of within-program analysis

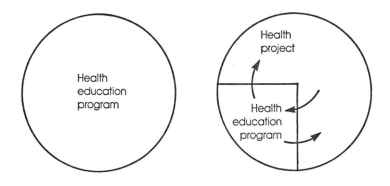

Where the program office is going to be located physically should influence planning. If the program is to operate out of the central organization office, flow of resources, communications, and access to key people will be facilitated. This location may, however, result in the program's being subjected to a degree of scrutiny and review not usual in a district office or other, more distant setting. Program leaders in close daily association with their superiors are also unlikely to have a great deal of freedom to exercise their own judgment. Another aspect of program-office location is the extent to which it is visible to the organization and the public. A prominent setting can foster awareness of a program's aims; it can foster resentment and resistance as well.

Another factor of consequence is the position the program occupies in the hierarchy. If a program is subordinate to many others, decision making may be impeded. Program planners who know ahead of time what the potential sources of difficulty are can take steps to minimize them.

Staffing is an overriding concern at the intraprogram level, because it is staff knowledge, competence, and personal interactions that determine to a great extent the success of a program. In this part of the analysis, one should consider participating health professionals in terms of their disciplines, skills, and tasks. Major differences in status or roles may negatively affect program coordination. The staff's knowledge of health education, their skills in delivering educational messages, and their sensitivity and ability to listen to others may limit success. Attitudes of the staff toward the consumers and toward each other are also important. Constructive, positive outlooks will help create a climate for success. Staff members should, of course, be used according to their skills. People who are dealing directly with consumers, for example, should be particularly effective in applying educational principles. Those who are to select and refer people into the program or to establish other relationships with other agencies or services should be highly skilled in communications.[3]

A final point regarding program personnel concerns the meshing of their various efforts. Some program designs call for several types of personnel to intervene with educational messages in a sequential manner. In these the messages must be coordinated but not the personnel. Other designs require a team effort in which team members can function interchangeably and all are familiar with the target population and the goals of the program. The planner should bear in mind the fact that the greater the amount of collaboration and coordination required, the more the time that must be spent in discussion, planning, and communication.[4]

Other factors important in the administrative diagnosis at the intraprogram level are space, funding, and support. Many times all a program needs is space—a desk, a clinic, a community hall. But this can be one of the most difficult requirements to fill. Similarly, funding may not be a factor, or it may occupy most of the program director's time. The larger the number of funding sources, the greater the amount of time that will have to be devoted to keeping them informed about program progress. Finally, if a program is not self-sufficient and is dependent on other departments or agencies for clerical, or, more generally, janitorial or security support, these matters deserve attention before the program is launched. Program implementation can be seriously hindered by staff who are not included in the orientation to the program.[5]

Within-Organization Analysis

The within-organization analysis is addressed to the interface between the health education program and the larger, sponsoring organization with all its other programs (fig. 7.3). The factors to be considered here are five: (1) relative newness of health education as part of the organization; (2) the degree to which health education is a known and valued form of intervention; (3) status; (4) effects of the program on other parts of the organization; and (5) readiness of the organization for change.

A new direction, especially if it represents the first time an organization has seriously undertaken health education, requires that special attention be given to interpreting the goals and function of health education generally and

FIGURE 7.3

The health education program as it relates to the sponsoring organization: Focus of within-organization analysis

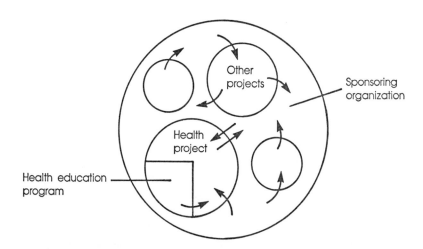

of the program specifically. It may be that special attention should also be directed to helping concerned health professionals learn to collaborate with health educators. These measures may not be necessary if the organization has had positive experiences with health education; on the other hand, negative experiences may have to be overcome. Depending on the organization's history in this regard, it may be receptive to fresh approaches, or it may be wary of new ideas.

It is important to try to make certain that everyone working with the program, at whatever level, use the term *health education* in the same way—to designate a planned, formal endeavor. Some health-care providers may be dubious of the worth of educational interventions and their potential for impact on a health problem. Recognition that health education is a legitimate and valid undertaking can be speeded if there is agreement on terminology. The planner soliciting support from key personnel should bear in mind the likelihood that some will be more open to the idea of health education than others.

The planner's status will affect his or her relationships with other personnel. Junior staff members do not behave in the same ways with superiors and with peers. Senior staff members will, of course, have greater authority and decision-making power. Consultants may have a different role altogether, devoting large amounts of time to promoting full understanding of and support for the program. If there are several co-equal program workers (as would be the case when each of several workers is responsible for a significant segment of a total program), then coordination among them is a prerequisite to coordination with the larger organization. Negotiations for resources, including good will and support, will be influenced by status also. A physician or top administrator may be more effective in such negotiations than a nurse, health educator, or social worker.

Some units and groups in the organization may see the introduction of a new program as a threat. Individuals may believe in the value of health education and feel that they have been providing an acceptable version, only to find that their efforts are apparently being criticized and discarded. Perhaps the new program alters patient flow and reduces patient loads in a clinic or adds to the burden of the receptionists. Perhaps it overlaps an already existing program. It is not difficult to imagine an agency's resisting a new program dealing with the elderly when it has been conducting a hot-meals program in the neighborhoods for several years. Sensitivity to the impact of a new program on other programs, services, and the like is important to the successful implementation of the new program. Anticipating possible negative reactions is crucial.

The opposite situation may also obtain. There may be great pockets of support throughout the organization, and the health education specialist may be overrun by enthusiastic staff members, each of whom has a long list of ideas. Learning to say no to well-meant demands while fanning continuing interest in educational interventions requires diplomacy as well as systematic planning.

Since the introduction of a new health education program within an organization is likely to meet the same resistance as previous innovations within the same system, it will be helpful if the planner has a reasonably good idea of the degree to which his or her organization is ready for change. General indicators of the readiness of an organization for change are listed in *Putting Knowledge to Use: A Distillation of the Literature Regarding Knowledge Transfer and Change.* They can be summarized as follows: The program must seem to be relatively *worthwhile* to those who have the decision and power to adopt it; that is, it must promise to be effective, it must appear to be generally more cost-effective than alternatives, and it must be relatively free of negative side effects. Further, the organization must be *able, willing,* and *informed* if the program is to be adopted and retained.[6]

One list of readiness indicators has been labeled AVICTORY. It provides for a more detailed assessment of readiness for change.

A = ability to carry out the change (capability, resources, and social costs)

V = values; compatibility with mission or goals

I = ideas or information about the qualities of the innovation (communicability, observability, susceptibility to successive modifications, divisibility, reversibility, scientific status)

C = circumstances that prevail at the time (climate of trust, willingness to entertain a challenge)

T = timing or readiness for consideration of the idea; early involvement of potential users

O = obligation or accepted need to deal with a particular problem; relevance, commitment; shared interest in solving recognized problems

R = resistance or inhibiting factors; skill in working through uncertainty and risks

Y = yield or perceived prospect of payoff for adoption; expected reward; belief in the efficiency of the innovation[7]

A rating scale or checklist based on a detailed list similar to AVICTORY can be devised for any organization. Such a checklist (see appendix D for an example) will be useful in pinpointing trouble spots and areas of potential problems and in assessing levels of knowledge and interest in various sectors of the organization.[8] One can note by this means where thorough information-sharing efforts are needed and which individuals important in terms of allocating resources require special attention. It should be remembered that having administrative approval does not ensure the complete cooperation of all those on whom the planner may depend for support.

How much support there is in an organization for a particular program may be related to the number and kinds of activities already under way. A major reorganization or a budget slash, for example, will surely have top organizational priority that will detract from health education concerns and drain attention away from the new program. Support can also be affected by dissimilarities in expectations for the program. Administrators may see the aims of a program in an entirely different light than program workers. Immediate results may seem desirable at the program level (to guarantee the support of a governing board, for example); while at the administrative level an extended developmental period may seem necessary. Discrepancies in pace or expectations regarding the rate of development and delivery can lead to difficulties.

Scrutinizing administrative policies is also part of the within-organization analysis. The planner will want to identify which policies of the organization dovetail with and support the needs of the program and which do not. Administrative, personnel, and patient-care standards of the organization should be compatible with the aims of the program. And there should be enough flexibility in the organization to accommodate necessary adaptations in record-keeping systems. Early attention to such details will reduce crises after the program is under way.

Finally, the planner should note the decision-making structure of the organization. Are there formal committees for approving different functions of the organization? How might this affect the program? Will new types of personnel be used in the program? Will patient-flow patterns be altered because of new types of activities? Will there be new patterns of interaction with community groups? Any such plans may require special organizational review and initial approval at more than one organizational level. And the review and approval process may have to be ongoing if different interventions are planned for different phases of the program.

Interorganizational Analysis

The interorganizational analysis investigates the extent to which the world outside the sponsoring organization may influence the orderly development of the program (fig. 7.4). Early in the analysis the planner should determine whether other agencies have been delivering similar services to the target population. Further, he or she should try to arrive at a clear idea of the kinds

FIGURE 7.4

The health education program as it relates to the community: Focus of interorganizational analysis

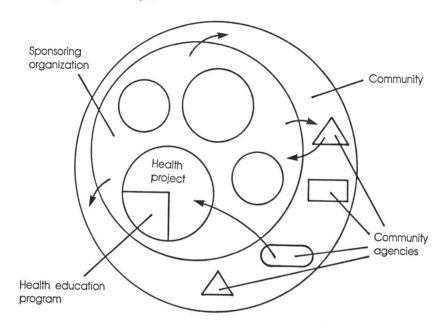

of coordination with other organizations and professionals that will be needed to ensure the success of the program. Timely communication and planning in this regard reduces resistance and eliminates stumbling blocks. More importantly, it results in fewer problems for the members of the target group.

If the health education program is heavily weighted toward the enabling factors, community-level assessment should be very thorough. If, on or types of personnel are involved, the planner should make sure that there are no regulations, legislation, or standards in conflict with his or her purposes. Conflicts of this sort occur only rarely, but they can be extremely disruptive. Secondly, if the health education program takes the organization beyond its usual and known mandate, it will be important to allow time for explaining the new activities to key groups, organizations, or individuals in the community. Again, change can be unnerving to some. It may be viewed as jeopardizing the stability of an organization. And it may trigger jurisdictional disputes that could interfere with program success. Having a hospital begin home visits to dying patients, a health department launch primary care programs, a community agency start a campaign to change automobile safety laws—all may be perceived as changes in mandates. When change is viewed as threatening, efforts should be made at the outset to allay anxieties and clear up misunderstandings.

If the health education program is heavily weighted toward the enabling factors, community-level assessment should be very thorough. If, on the other hand, the program is within the usual mandate of the organization and is directed toward the usual target population with little change expected in the activities of the population, the planner probably will not need to give much attention to community factors. Whether the program is more or less directed toward enabling factors will depend on the relative importance and changeability of such factors as determined in the educational diagnosis. If the educational diagnosis revealed major problems of transportation and baby-sitting for women who were expected to appear for prenatal care, then the administrative diagnosis must look beyond the organization providing prenatal care to other organizations that might help with transportation and child care.

SUMMARY

The purpose of an administrative diagnosis is to identify administrative and organizational factors that might facilitate or impede successful implementation of a health education program. The goal of the diagnosis is to reduce to a minimum those factors that might prevent a soundly conceived program from achieving its full and positive impact. Realities of the organization, the community, and of professional practice must be considered in order to minimize negative impacts and maximize the potential benefits to the program.

Steps in the administrative diagnosis include an assessment of available resources, an explicit allocation of those resources in the forms of a budget and a timetable, and a determination of hierarchical and cooperative relations between the personnel and resources within the health education program; between health education and the broader health program in which it serves; between these and the broader organization or institution sponsoring them; and between all of these and the larger community of organizations in which they operate.

EXERCISES

1.   Identify the resources required for your program with a specific budget and timetable or PERT chart.

2. Analyze how your program would affect and be affected by other programs and units within a health agency or educational institution.

3. Describe the interorganizational coordination that would be required to achieve the objectives of your program.

8

Evaluation and the Accountable Practitioner

THE ACCOUNTABLE HEALTH EDUCATOR cultivates an attitude toward professional practice which ensures that every new population or patient is approached diagnostically and that every program is developed as an experiment. The need for evaluation will be understood by the practitioner who has applied the diagnostic steps up to this point and has found great gaps in the scientific and professional literature on the effectiveness of educational methods applied to specific behavioral problems in specific types of populations. If one can not provide assurance on the basis of prior research, one must evaluate to be accountable.

We define *evaluation* simply as the comparison of an object of interest against a standard of acceptability. Objects of interest in health education include, at one end of the PRECEDE framework, the long-range goals of improved quality of life or health and social benefits. At the other end, objects of interest include the activities, methods, materials, and programs of health ed-

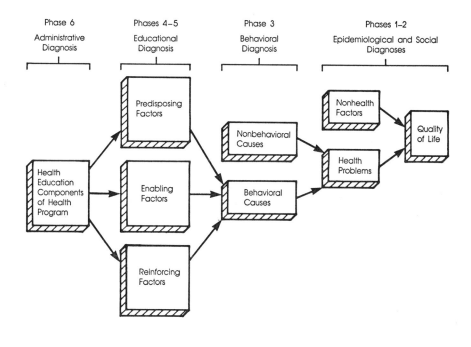

Phase 6	Phases 4–5	Phase 3	Phases 1–2
Administrative Diagnosis	Educational Diagnosis	Behavioral Diagnosis	Epidemiological and Social Diagnoses

Predisposing Factors

Nonhealth Factors

Quality of Life

Health Education Components of Health Program

Enabling Factors

Nonbehavioral Causes

Health Problems

Behavioral Causes

Reinforcing Factors

ucation. All the intermediate effects of health education, including changes in predisposing, enabling, and reinforcing factors and achievement of behavioral objectives, are also objects of interest. This chapter will describe the levels of evaluation appropriate to these various objects of interest and several designs that can be used to compare them against standards of acceptability.

In previous chapters, we have worked from right to left along the causal chain implied by the PRECEDE framework. It was a systematic search for the root causes holding the greatest promise of yielding social or health benefits assuming that health education activities and resources can effectively change those root causes. Evaluation, as described in this chapter, applies the same logic and framework as applied to diagnosis in the preceding chapters, except that the order of attention is from left to right, from immediate activities and resources to ultimate health outcomes and social benefits. Evaluation verifies the diagnosis after the program has begun. If the objectives for social, health, behavioral, and educational effects of the program have been well written, the objects of interest and the standards of acceptability are already identified.

LEVELS OF EVALUATION

There are three levels at which a health education program can be evaluated. It can be evaluated in terms of process, in terms of impact, and in terms of outcome (fig. 8.1). In a process evaluation, the object of interest is professional practice, and the standard of acceptability is appropriate practice. Quality is monitored by various means, including audit, peer review, accreditation, certification, and government or administrative surveillance of contracts and grants. Standards of acceptability are established both professionally and administratively and are derived chiefly by means of consensus among health education specialists.

The second level is impact evaluation. Evaluation here focuses on the immediate impact the program (or some aspect of it) has on knowledge, attitudes, and behavior. Have the predisposing, enabling, and reinforcing factors that influence the health-related behavior been altered? Have the short-term goals of a program been met? In terms of behavior, the planner will ask such questions as: Does it take as long for members of the target population to seek medical care as it did before the program? Is there an increase in health-enhancing behavior? Are diseases being diagnosed earlier? Has exposure to risk been reduced? Cost-effectiveness is the most succinct standard of acceptability in impact evaluation.

At the third level, the level of outcome evaluation, the objects of interest are mortality and morbidity. Have the incidence and prevalence of the condition(s) been affected by a program? Have the rate and length of survival

FIGURE 8.1

Three levels of evaluation in relation to the PRECEDE framework

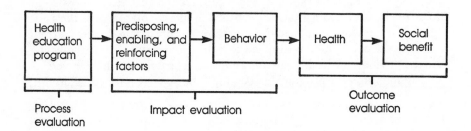

following detection and treatment changed? Again, cost-effectiveness is one standard of acceptability; this standard can be expressed more humanely in terms of number of lives saved or improved. Outcome evaluation is a long-term undertaking requiring large population samples.

When the number of educational booklets distributed is the measure of success, one is using a process measure of evaluation. The number of patients who made appointments or showed up at cancer screening centers is an impact-evaluation statement. Years later, outcome might be measured in terms of increased survival and reduced mortality and morbidity.

At this point in the history of patient, school, occupational, and community health education, impact evaluation rather than outcome or process evaluation is most needed. Currently, for a number of reasons, it is not efficient to focus exclusively on process. Physicians, nurses, and other health professionals are not uniformly ready for more intensive examination of their skills and effectiveness in patient education, for example. Even if they were, evaluators are not quite sure what the standards of acceptability for communication with patients should be. It has not yet been possible to translate standards of educational practice in many clinical and community settings into hard criteria for purposes of process evaluation. In addition to the problem of defining criteria, a number of practitioners, including physicians, feel burdened and sometimes threatened by peer review and government surveillance. In community and patient education, then, process evaluation is not the most fruitful pursuit. In school health education, there is a stronger data base for the assessment of communication behavior. Classroom teaching practices have customarily been subjected to intense scrutiny.

It is also premature to expect most programs in their present state of development to have measurable outcomes. Evidence linking specific behaviors to specific medical or health results is still somewhat tenuous. And in some cases health-related behavior is not sufficiently established as medically effective. Breast self-examination is one such behavior; restricting cholesterol intake is another. The possible benefits of these practices are not well established. Further, successfully changing a behavior may have negative consequences. For example, a patient may be encouraged to take a prescribed drug, which turns out to have side effects. These the patient ignores because the physician failed to identify the other drugs or foods the patient was taking.

Another difficulty with emphasizing outcome evaluation in most community and school programs is that such evaluation can not be done efficiently. Health outcomes and social benefits often do not appear for long periods of time, and populations rarely remain stable. An evaluation of education and community organization efforts directed toward cancer control in terms of reduced morbidity and mortality, for example, would require greater resources, larger populations, and more follow-up time than are likely to be available in those programs.

DESIGNS FOR EVALUATION

At this stage in the development of health education, impact evaluation, the assessment of the changes in knowledge, attitudes, beliefs, and, especially, behavior that come about as a result of health education programs, is the level of evaluation most likely to produce the greatest improvements in such programs.

Evaluation can be done according to a number of different designs, ranging from the simple but often neglected collection of routine data on an ongoing basis to the collection of data in highly rigorous, highly controlled experimental settings. The historical, record-keeping approach, the simplest, is applicable to most programs; the controlled experimental approach will usually be impractical. Each has its own utility. Practitioners will make their selections based on the kinds of data desired and the uses to which the data will be put. All the designs can be implemented in two or three steps.

Design A: The Historical, Record-Keeping Approach

Design A, the record-keeping approach, yields charts and graphs that effectively demonstrate what is occurring in a program or community. The procedure is simple. The first step is to construct a dummy graph showing the expected relationship between inputs and outcomes. The second step is to set up a record-keeping procedure to accumulate the data. The last step is to calculate and chart the data periodically, plotting the direction and magnitude of change taking place over time. How often should one tabulate and chart the data? That depends on the number of times the events being tabulated occur.

An example of a design-A graph is given in figure 8.2. It demonstrates the sequential benefits of different educational approaches during three phases of a program conducted by a venereal disease clinic over a two-year-plus period. The impact of each educational strategy can be noted both in changes in the absolute number of patients appearing at the clinic and in the composition of the patient population. The change in interviewing policy (C) was a change from asking patients to identify their sexual contacts to encouraging them to take the responsibility for seeing that their sexual partners received treatment. The behavioral impact in terms of the male/female ratio of patients at this point was most notable.[1] The ratios (looked at in combination with the graph) show increases in females and whites using the clinic until

FIGURE 8.2

Visits to a venereal disease clinic, by month

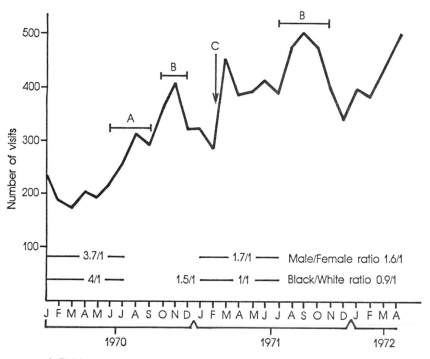

A Field-worker contacting street groups

B Use of radio spots

C Change in interviewing policy

SOURCE: Reproduced with permission of the author and publisher from Atwater, John B: "Adapting the Venereal Disease Clinic to Today's Problem." **American Journal of Public Health** 64: 433–437, May 1974.

1972 when the numbers were close to equal. Other examples are listed in the bibliography.[2]

Design B: The "Stop-Everything," Inventory Approach

The inventory approach, which we are labeling design B, requires making a special effort periodically to collect data. Sometimes the prevailing record-keeping system does not incorporate the data required, and changing the system, perhaps expanding it, would be too disruptive to the service program.

Rather than accumulating the data on an ongoing basis, as is done with design A, one can obtain the data by conductig special surveys.

First the evaluator sets target dates for the assessments. Then he or she identifies the expected target levels. Finally he or she takes the surveys as a way of estimating the levels achieved at the selected points in time. Literature that provides examples of the inventory approach is listed in the chapter notes.[3]

For some kinds of programs, such as smoking-cessation programs, the critical points for measuring behavior are highly standardized. A review of the literature will reveal the times at which people are likeliest to drop out or backslide in programs dealing with such problems as smoking, antibiotic therapy, and oral contraceptive use.

Design C: The Comparative, "How We Stack Up Against Others," Approach

Evaluation by means of the comparative approach is an extension of the inventory or record-keeping approach. The same procedures are followed, except that new data are introduced. (1) One can usually identify similar data on programs in other places; (2) borrow or copy the record forms used in these programs or buy into a common, standardized format for collecting data or keeping records on the similar programs; and (3) do periodic comparisons between the programs on the same basis as design A or design B.

Various kinds of national data are available. For example, the National Health Survey provides data derived from standardized questionnaires that can be compared with data collected in local programs. National norms suggest what health educators can expect in relation to breast examination, Pap smears, smoking cessation, and other health behaviors. Comparability is an essential feature of cumulative evaluation. For this reason we recommend using standardized formats for collecting data rather than developing original questionnaires. Examples of the comparative or normative approach can be found in the literature.[4]

Design D: The Controlled-Comparison, Quasi-Experimental, Approach

In the controlled-comparison approach, an evaluator first identifies a community or population similar to the target population but one not receiving the program. He or she then applies design A or B in both the program being evaluated and the comparison program and periodically compares the two communities. One might want to compare the effects of various kinds of interventions in similar populations, in schools, for example, or in communities. The Stanford three-community study is the most notable contemporary example of the latter application.[5] Three communities were studied, one in which an intensive all-out educational effort had been made, another in which only a mass media effort was made, and another in which neither effort was made, although there were comparable resources and facilities. The effectiveness of the strategies used in each of the three experimental communities and their various subpopulations was compared using impact data from surveys. Other examples of this approach can be found in the literature.[6]

Design E: The Controlled-Experimental Approach

The controlled-experimental approach is comparable to the clinical trial in medical studies. It requires a formal procedure for random assignment of individuals within the target population to two (and sometimes more) groups. If there are two, one group will receive the educational treatment and one will not. It should be noted that in this approach it must be possible to deny certain people the treatment. Once the groups are set up and the program is under way, the evaluator uses approach A or approach B for both the experimental and the control groups. Baseline data may be collected on all groups, but this is not essential. Records or survey data over time are then graphed to see how the groups compare at various points in the treatment.[7] Smoking-cessation programs are often evaluated according to design E.

Design F: The Evaluative Research Project

The most complex of the evaluation designs, what might be described as a full-scale evaluative research project, is unlikely to be feasible in most community programs. Procedures are similar to those for design E, the controlled-experimental approach, except that multiple groups are randomized in factorial designs, and multiple measures are obtained on intermediate variables such as changes in knowledge, attitudes, and skills as well as on outcomes and impact variables such as behavior and health. Group tendencies are analyzed as are intragroup effects. The design can accommodate numerous refinements. Programs consisting of as many as six different treatments applied to various subgroups within randomized groups can be evaluated by means of this design.[8]

Somewhere between the simplicity of design A with its inconclusive but suggestive findings and the complexity of Design F with its headaches is a level of evaluation that is feasible and practicable as well as rigorous. The problem with the more complicated designs is that they usually have to be carried out under highly controlled conditions, which makes the behavioral circumstances unusual or unnatural.[9] Often it is necessary to remove people from their social milieu, the ordinary context for their behavior. Finding willing participants for controlled, randomized experiments is seldom easy. Further, such designs require informed consent.

In short, what one gains in internal validity through the more rigorous randomized procedures one may sacrifice in feasibility and in generalizability of findings. Can data from highly controlled classroom or clinical facilities be generalized to private practice and community based programs?[10] The only way to answer this question is to continue to accumulate data in different settings, evaluating programs and methods as they are developed according to careful educational diagnoses.

SUMMARY

In this brief chapter we attempt only to introduce some concepts and approaches to evaluation that have particular utility in health education today, considering the weak scientific base on which many educational decisions will have to be made. The concept of accountability in the practice of health education should lead the conscientious educator to approach each program as an experiment. As in a laboratory experiment, the results of a health education program represent the impact or outcomes of an experimental manipulation of some input or process that has been hypothesized to have a positive effect on those outcomes. If the effect is found, the hypothesis is confirmed, and the educational, behavioral, or administrative diagnosis is verified.

Several designs for evaluation are described in simple steps, and numerous examples of each are cited in the reference notes. This brief introduction to evaluation and the references cited can serve as a springboard for further study of evaluation methods, not as a sufficient guide in itself for those without experience.

The five levels of evaluation begin with the simple record-keeping approach, in which routinely collected data are accumulated and tabulated periodically to show progress or achievement of expected goals. In the second level, one does not depend on routinely collected data; instead, one carries out special surveys periodically. Both of these approaches provide historical comparisons. In the remaining levels of evaluation design, one adds to these basic data-collection procedures one or more comparison groups, either in another population receiving a similar program or in the same population (comparing those who receive the health education with those who do not). The latter designs are considered the strongest for scientific purposes, but the "lower-level" designs are adequate and necessary for routine evaluation.

EXERCISES

1. What are the objects of interest and standards of acceptability in your objectives from previous exercises?

2. Which evaluation design would you use if you had limited resources? If you had unlimited resources? If there were no other programs of the kind you are conducting to compare with?

3. Propose an evaluation plan for your program, indicating the data to be collected, the procedures for collection and tabulation of the data, and the comparisons you expect to be able to make. Use charts or graphs with hypothetical data.

9

PRECEDE Applied to School Health Education

HEALTH EDUCATION OCCURS in virtually every setting in which there is human interaction. It is practiced by an increasing variety of people whose experience and training varies both in emphasis and in rigor. * While some health educators are professionals with advanced degrees in public health, education, nursing, medicine, and behavioral sciences, others have considerably less training as, for example, nonprofessional aides recruited for grass-roots health education efforts in inner-city neighborhoods, rural areas, or the work place.[1]

---

*The apparent inconsistencies in the professional preparation and practice for health education in the United States have led recently to formal discussions aimed at delineating the roles, functions, and competencies required for proficiency in health education. These activities constitute a first step toward the establishment of certifica-

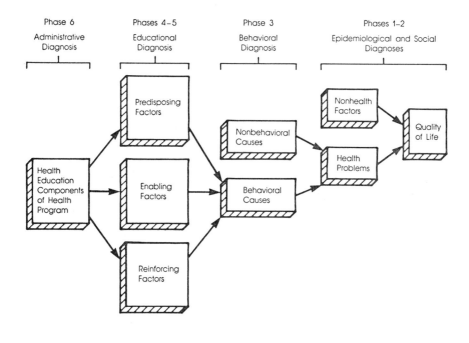

Phase 6	Phases 4–5	Phase 3	Phases 1–2
Administrative Diagnosis	Educational Diagnosis	Behavioral Diagnosis	Epidemiological and Social Diagnoses

Recognizing the many settings in which health education can occur, the purpose of this chapter and the next is to illustrate how the PRECEDE framework might be applied in two areas in which health education is especially pervasive: public schools and patient-care practice. The application of the PRECEDE planning approach in these two markedly different kinds of settings demonstrates the practical value and potential generalizability of the framework.

tion procedures and competency assurance in health education. (See *Preparation and Practice of Community, Patient, and School Health Educators: Proceedings of the Workshop on Commonalities and Differences* Hyattsville, Md.: Division of Associated Health Professions, Bureau of Health Manpower, Health Resources Administration, 1978.)

REVIEW OF SCHOOL HEALTH EDUCATION

To put in perspective the potential applications of PRECEDE in school health education planning, a brief review of school health education in general and curriculum development in particular may be helpful. There is much variation in the way health education is offered in schools, and this variation seems to stem largely from policies at the individual school and district level as well as from mandates in statewide education codes.[2] In some instances health education is offered as a unit of study within a course in biology, home economics, physical education, or behavioral science. In others it is offered as health education in an independent semester or term course. Few school districts provide comprehensive health education in each grade from kindergarten to twelfth grade; most offerings are sporadic, at selected grade levels only.

Although some schools offer educational programs that attempt to intervene in specific health behavior problems such as smoking, weight control, and dental health, the majority offer health education as a phase in a general curriculum plan. In educational parlance, *curriculum development* generally refers to the systematic selection of goals, content, teaching methods and materials, and evaluation procedures for a given topic of study. Curriculum planning in schools is typically a committee function, ideally taking into account suggestions and concerns of parents, community representatives, and students as well as faculty and administration. For informative overviews of traditional curriculum planning in school health education we recommend the work of Russell, Bruess and Gay, and Sorensen and Bender.

Two national projects on school health curriculum stand out in the literature. The first was the School Health Education Study (SHES), a monumental undertaking* initiated in the early 1960s; the other is the School Health Curriculum Project (SHCP) initiated in 1974. The SHES curriculum, which was representative of a very detailed and complex national design effort, was based on the philosophic and theoretical importance of interplay among three fundamental concepts: growing and developing, interaction, and decision making. Its emphasis was on basic general concepts rather than on specific *topics* and *problems*.[3] Paradoxically, the philosophical and conceptual strength of the SHES curriculum may have been its major weakness. Many health educators apparently found it difficult to understand and apply in the classroom situation.[4]

The School Health Curriculum Project (SHCP), unlike the SHES approach, was initiated as a specific effort. Its original focus was on educating

---

*Although conducted as a national project, the SHES curriculum was not intended to be a guide for nationwide implementation; rather, it was a conceptual guide to be adapted at the local levels.

children about the dangerous effects of cigarette smoking; that focus has since become more comprehensive.

> The importance of the Project [SHCP] for disease prevention nationally was first recognized by the National Clearinghouse for Smoking and Health. The Project showed potential for educating students about the health consequences of the personal decision to smoke. But the Project is bigger than any one health topic: It is about the whole body and the biological, cultural, and social factors that influence it; it is an experiential curriculum developed to facilitate individual understanding of and responsibility for health.[5]

To date, the SHCP curriculum has been developed for grades three through seven with a specific focus in each grade on various health concepts and behaviors as they relate to a given body system. An elaborate teacher-training component is available for the project with an emphasis on experiential teaching methods and management of health education "learning centers."[6]

Even though there is evidence in the literature of philosophically sound curricula that include imaginative teaching strategies, the benefits, beyond short-term knowledge and attitude change, continue to go largely undetected. Kunstel has suggested that one of the important missing links in the curriculum development and implementation process has been the failure to identify the needs of the local community served by school health education programs.[7] The chances for positive educational outcomes diminish when curricular plans fail to take into account community needs. The assessment of these needs seems to be critical, and it is in this connection that the PRECEDE framework can be helpful.

USING PRECEDE TO PLAN SCHOOL HEALTH EDUCATION

Needs assessment is often only nominally a part of educational planning approaches. In cases in which it is not overlooked entirely, it is replaced by reference to national or state norms, which may have no bearing on local needs. What often happens in school health education is that sound curriculum planning is relinquished in favor of adopting a textbook or transplanting a national curriculum to the local level.

Recommendations to begin curriculum planning with a thorough needs assessment parallel the first two phases of the PRECEDE process (discussed in chaps. 2 and 3). Those phases consist of identifying and ranking the social problems (the social/quality of life diagnosis) and health problems (the epidemiological diagnosis) of a given target population. The value of this approach is reinforced by Kunstel, who offers three reasons for assessing community needs. The first has to do with establishing appropriate goals and objectives: "Choices must be made about what should be included and what should be left out." The second has to do with specificity of program purpose: "Teachers can more effectively carry out instruction when they understand why particular content and activity are included." The third is political: "Parents may be more supportive of the inclusion of controversial content when a need has been clearly established and communicated."[7]

THE SOCIAL AND EPIDEMIOLOGICAL DIAGNOSES

Social and epidemiological diagnoses for school health education planning would be more useful if it included both the general community and the school community. Although amplifying the diagnoses in this way will take more time and effort, the benefits are well worth it. Knowing what the health problems in the community are can give significant insight into the relative importance of problems in the school setting. As in any program planning endeavor, every effort should be made to have representation from all groups that will be affected. For school health education, the committee should at least include students, parents, teachers, administrators, and community health professionals. Both the attention to broader community health issues and the representation of people from the community will make school health planning more responsive to the needs and concerns of the population that supports the school.

A hypothetical example will help illustrate the point. Suppose both social and epidemiological diagnoses were conducted by a curriculum committee for a target community served by ten elementary schools, four junior high schools, and two senior high schools. Let us say that a social diagnosis revealed that the major social problems were: inflation (especially food and health-care costs), unemployment, absenteeism, and an increase in the crime rate, especially among juveniles. An epidemiological diagnosis rendered an extensive list of health problems, presented in table 9.1.

As the committee examined and compared the reported social and health problems, it found that cardiovascular diseases and problem drinking accounted for approximately 80 percent of workdays lost (absenteeism). It was noted that medical treatment and care for cardiovascular problems and accidents combined as the major cause for increases in medical costs in the community. Finding such linkages between social problems and health prob-

TABLE 9.1
Health problems (alphabetically listed) identified at community level

Problem	Basis for identification as problem
Accidents	Industrial and auto accidents rank as the second leading cause of death for all ages. Accidents in general are the leading cause of death for people aged two through twenty-four.
Cardiovascular diseases	Total number of patients reported to have cardiovascular disease has risen 25 percent in last five years while population has increased only 12 percent.
Dental health	Local dental society has released figures indicating that the adult rates for decayed, missing, and filled teeth have risen 20 percent in last decade.
Emotional health	Community mental health services indicate increase in the number of people seeking help. Much of the increase is associated with alcohol-related problems.
Hypertension	Although there have been only slight increases in incidence rates, rates in the three-county area of which this community is a part have traditionally been well above the national average.
Teenage pregnancies	There is a good deal of community concern over the fact that the incidence of teenage, out-of-wedlock pregnancies has increased consistent with reported national averages.

lems is essential if there is to be any relationship between health education efforts and health outcomes and social benefits.

With data from the community in hand, the committee repeats the process at the school level. It uses, in addition to existing school attendance, health, and academic records, interview, questionnaire, and small-group methods to gather input from parents, students, and school personnel. Results of the diagnoses are presented in tables 9.2 and 9.3.

As it did in the community analysis, the committee studies the school data to see if linkages exist between social and health problems. Although the associations between the two sets of problems turn out to be, in most cases, tenuous, some are quite suggestive. For example, it might be hypothesized that a program reducing the incidence of tobacco, alcohol, and drug use will

TABLE 9.2

Social problems identified within the school community

School personnel and parents

> Inadequate budget (E, J, H)
> Overcrowding in classrooms (J, H)
> Absenteeism and tardiness due to "cutting school" (J, H)
> Vandalism (J, H)
> Alienation among some social groups (J, H)
> Availability and sale of tobacco, alcohol, drugs (E, J, H)
> Student scores on achievement tests below state and national average (H)
> Inadequate indoor play facilities in some schools (E)
> Questionable competence of some school personnel (E, J, H)
> Increase in incidence of teenage pregnancies (H)

Students

> Not enough parking space for students (H)
> Prejudice in some teachers (J, H)
> Gymnasiums not kept open at nights and on weekends for recreation (J, H)
> Some teachers' and administrators' letting kids "get away with too much" (J, H)
> Cafeteria food not very good (E, J, H)

NOTE: E—elementary level; J—junior high level; H—senior high level.

have an impact not only on the sale of these substances in schools but on absenteeism, tardiness, vandalism, and school performance as well. Again, the important point is that in taking the time for social and epidemiological diagnoses, the curriculum committee has made it possible to identify problems that subsequent programs *may* be able to affect. Traditionally, changes in short-term knowledge, attitudes, and skills have been the only discernible changes resulting from educational intervention.

A comparison of the health problems reported at the community and school levels (table 9.4) reveals some interesting similarities. Accidents, dental health problems, teenage pregnancies, problem drinking, and emotional problems, common in both communities, are prime candidates for subsequent program focus. Further, since hypertension has been a rather long standing problem seemingly indigenous to the area and since the incidence of cardiovascular disease is increasing, health education efforts aimed at minimizing associated risk factors would be appropriate. Obesity, cigarette smoking, emotional stress—all problems at the school level—merit serious attention in this regard.

TABLE 9.3

Health problems identified by an epidemiological diagnosis of the school community

	Basis for identification as problem
Elementary schools	
Accidents	High frequency of preventable playground injuries and bicycle crashes.
Junior high schools	
Accidents	Playground injuries, sports mishaps, classroom experiments, fighting.
Dental health	Marked increase in various lesions.
Obesity	Survey recently conducted by a local university revealed that 35 percent of the area teenagers were overweight (not necessarily obese).
Tobacco, alcohol, drug use	Incidence according to records of counselors, school nurses, and police reports is up in all three categories over comparable records five years ago.
Senior high schools	
Accidents	Same as junior high with addition of automobile mishaps.
Tobacco, alcohol, drug use	Same as junior high except high prevalence.
Obesity	Same as junior high.
Dental health	Same as junior high plus a noted increase in gingivitis.
Emotional health	Counselors report an increase in number of students who are seeking assistance for emotional problems related to family and personal stress and alcohol- drug-related problems.
Teenage pregnancy	Incidence of teenage, out-of-wedlock pregnancies has increased 20 percent in last five years.

TABLE 9.4

Comparison of health problems (alphabetically listed) at the community and school levels

Community	School (all grades combined)
Accidents	Accidents
Cardiovascular diseases	Alcohol and drug use and abuse
Dental health	Dental health
Emotional health (mostly related to problem drinking)	Emotional problems
Hypertension	Teenage pregnancy
Teenage pregnancy	Vision and hearing

The utility of social and epidemiological diagnoses in school health education and the value of including community concerns and community representation in the planning of school health education should both be clear. By means of these steps, the interest and support of the community in program implementation will be increased.

BEHAVIOR CHANGE AS A GOAL IN SCHOOLS

It should be obvious that the process implied in the PRECEDE framework is impossible without identification of health problems within a given target population. However, problem identification is just the first step. Once problems have been identified—and rated in terms of importance and changeability—it is necessary to identify the behaviors that may be linked to the health problem(s) in question. This is the behavioral diagnosis. That health education is inseparably related to health behavior is a primary assumption of the PRECEDE framework. But establishing cause-and-effect chains in human behavior is difficult even under the most carefully controlled circumstances using the most sophisticated multivariate analysis. The number of variables in play in the school and home environment, for example, is almost infinite. This, taken with the short-term nature of most opportunities for evaluation of school health education, makes it virtually impossible to tie classroom activities directly to health behaviors that show up over time.

While there is evidence that change in health behavior is a feasible and appropriate criterion for evaluation of patient and some community health education, practically no such evidence exists for health education in the school. Health behavior is so complex that it is likely the interplay of variables, not single forces, that shapes health outcomes. An educational experience is only one of the many factors that might make up the total picture of any person's health behavior. Recent studies on educational interventions for hypertension control corroborate the notion. In sum, recognizing the classroom limitations of health education in most schools, we would do well not to infer cause when the behavior is remote.

An emphasis on behavior change in the school setting is in fact somewhat misleading. There are of course occasions when teachers should be alert to specific behaviors such as poor dietary, dental health, or general hygiene practices. But the primary goal of most school health education efforts appears to be the maintenance of health-enhancing behaviors. In the case of smoking, for example, rare instances notwithstanding, teachers in kindergarten through fifth grade should surely be more concerned with factors related to the decision to smoke or not to smoke than with smoking-cessation strategies.

To establish immediate behavior change as the criterion for success in school health education would be technically and politically naïve. Taken to the extreme, such a policy might lead to unfair decisions about accountability. Suppose that behavioral criteria were established for all areas of the curriculum. Social studies and civics teachers might then be held accountable not only for their students' understanding of the democratic process and procedures in voting, but also for their voting records. "I'm sorry, Ms. Jones, we can't renew your contract. We've done a study and found that only 5 percent of your former students voted in the last election." To take another example, English teachers are commonly expected to help students master the skills of reading and writing. They are expected, further, to enhance the motivation of their pupils to read and write; and, except in special cases, it is thought that they should be held accountable for "passing" students who cannot read or write. But it is extremely doubtful that English teachers and their programs should be held accountable if students who have developed reading skills *choose* not to use them as adults.

EVALUATION

Evaluators of school health education, quite clearly, face a dilemma. On the one hand, they must hypothesize that health education in the school affects health practices, for how else can they justify the time and resources spent on it? On the other hand, it has not yet been possible to evaluate changes in behavior—the most desirable, logical, and convincing confirmation of the behavior hypothesis.

Add to this dilemma the observation that in most schools health education has not had adequate resources and has not been considered of first importance. Even if opportunities were available to evaluate behavioral outcomes, the results might be discouraging. These observations suggest a set of propositions that have implications for the development and support of school health education in the future:

1. School health education is pervasive but inadequately supported, organized, or delivered.
2. Because it is pervasive, it has the potential to affect the health of large numbers of people.
3. Because of inadequate support, organization, and delivery, that potential has been unrealized or undetected.
4. Efforts to determine the effects of school health education in terms of health improvements or behavior change are likely to be discouraging because:
   a) programs are inadequately supported, organized, or delivered.
   b) special evaluation procedures are needed to detect the effects.
5. Accordingly, the appropriate development and evaluation of school health education will be dependent in the short run on increased support and organization and in the long run on special evaluation research conducted over time.
6. Support and delivery require clarification of the goals, methods, and immediate impact of school health education. Process evaluation of teaching practice is needed, followed by short-run assessments of knowledge and skills.
7. Special evaluation research needed to determine long-term effects and social benefits from school health education will require governmental support.

These propositions suggest that school health education should be evaluated at the three levels discussed in chapter 8. The first level is process evaluation, in which standards of acceptability are defined by the profession in terms of organizational and teaching practice. The second level, impact evaluation, refers to the evaluation of the immediate effects of programs, evaluation that is done during the programs or at their conclusions. At the third level, outcome evaluation, is the assessment of health practices or behaviors that have been hypothesized to show up over the long term. Figure 9.1 illustrates the relationship between these various levels of evaluation and improved health education. Limited resources will dictate emphasis on process

FIGURE 9.1

Breaking the "poverty cycle" of health education

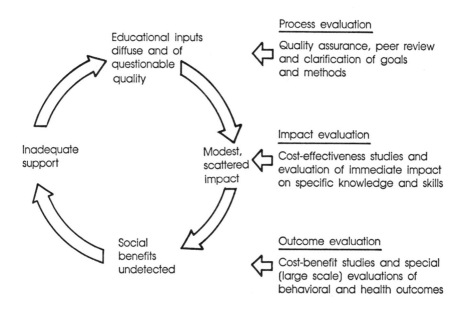

SOURCE: Adapted with permission from M. W. Kreuter and L. W. Green, "Evaluation of School Health Education: Identifying Purpose, Keeping Perspective," **Journal of School Health** 48 (April 1978): 228–35.

evaluation and, perhaps, in sequence, impact evaluation. As resources expand, it will be possible to develop procedures for outcome evaluation.

Though the need for all levels of evaluation is pressing, impact evaluation is currently, as we have noted, the most practical. Two characteristics of impact evaluation are worth emphasizing. First, such evaluation is immediate. The factors most often assessed at this level are usually identified during or immediately after a program. These typically include such learner variables as changes in knowledge, attitudes, beliefs, and skills, frequently assessed in relationship to the teaching strategies used. Second, impact evaluation is economical in terms of time and money; and it can be conducted with minimum inconvenience to the instructional program.

Impact evaluation pertains to the intermediate objectives of school health education: (1) the mastery of factual health-related information and (2) the development of selected skills, the application of which is associated with health-enhancing behavior.

KNOWLEDGE AND SKILLS AS THE GOALS IN SCHOOLS

Some contend that knowledge has little impact on health outcomes, but there is evidence that the association between knowledge and health is more than a philosophic one. For example, a well-controlled study of a random sample of 4,328 Maryland residents followed over an eight-year period, controlling for other socioeconomic factors, showed that lower death rates for arteriosclerosis; rheumatic heart disease; cancer of the lung, liver, and bile ducts; thromboembolism; chronic bronchitis; emphysema; and kidney disease were significantly associated with increased years of schooling.[8]

One can not imply that these differences are owing entirely to accumulations of knowledge. On the other hand, it is unlikely that there is no connection. A balanced perspective suggests that knowledge more than likely makes some of the difference. It increases decision-making ability and other skills required for effective living in a complex world. This, indeed, is the special contribution school health education can make to improved quality of life.

Health-related skills, whatever the setting in which they are taught, are viewed, in the PRECEDE framework, as enabling factors. Mastery of such skills increases the probability that students will use them to their health advantage. Depending on the grade level, students might be taught "to know their bodies,"[9] relaxation responses,[10] skills cited in the Health Activities Project,[11] the self-care approach,[12] as well as the more traditional hygiene practices typically offered in the schools. Emphasis on skill development leads to the opportunity for students to apply the knowledge they have been taught.[13]

When we assert that knowledge gain and the development of health-related skills are the important objectives of school health education at the impact level, we are not implying that these should be the sole focus of evaluation and evaluation-related research. We do strongly suggest, however, that their demonstration should constitute minimum standards of acceptability for the efficacy of school health education programs. Beyond that, there are numerous possibilities for useful evaluative research at this level. For example, to what extent should health education curricula be tailored to specific community or cultural idiosyncrasies? Although we have some indication that innovative curricula such as the School Health Curriculum Project and Health Activation[14] are effective, what impact do they have on family interest and involvement in the schools?[15]

Sometimes,. within the scope of the curriculum, research in the behavioral realm for situation-specific programs may be appropriate. Weight loss, smoking cessation, stress management, and physical fitness are typical examples of such programs.

HEALTH SKILLS IN **PRECEDE**

A basic question in school health education is: What outcomes are teachers to be held accountable for? Since schools serve communities it is only logical to suggest that school activities and teachers are primarily accountable to community members, especially parents. Parents should reasonably be able to expect their children, on completing a given grade, to have an adequate command of the necessary skills to successfully participate in the next grade. If fifth-grade pupils are supposed to be able to read at a certain rate and comprehend at a certain level, valid tests should be devised to ascertain those competencies. In health education, such tests would provide both short-range evaluation of impact and evidence that progress has been made toward enabling future behavior conducive to health.

The point was made earlier that school health educators, unlike patient health educators, are faced with the problem of linking health education activities to future behaviors, a problem confounded by the potential multitude of variables intervening over time. We believe that the PRECEDE framework can be useful in attacking this problem, particularly if the framework is modified. Recall the middle section of the framework, in which the relationship between health problems, health behaviors, and the constellation of factors antecedent to the behaviors is schematized. The suggested modification consists of allowing for *intermediate* outcomes by establishing objectives that interpose between the predisposing, enabling, and reinforcing factors contributing to a given behavior and the behavior itself (fig. 9.2). We have labeled these intermediate outcomes "health skills."

This modification in the PRECEDE framework has already been applied by several innovative researchers. Evans and his colleagues[16] and McAlister[17] have studied the effects of health education strategies designed to: (1) help children recognize the social pressures to smoke and (2) teach them assertiveness skills to cope with and resist those pressures. The results of their work suggest that teaching students assertiveness skills is effective in delaying the onset of smoking. From the point of view of health education planning, this interesting application of McGuire's "innoculation effect"[18] was conceptualized only after a careful consideration of predisposing factors (students' recognition of social pressures), enabling factors (students' lack of coping skills), and reinforcing factors (persuasion by peers and mass media).

How are students to demonstrate achievement at the health-skills level? By showing that they are in command of selected health-related information, that they have mastered certain physical skills (as in self-care skills), and that they have developed coping skills (as in assertiveness or decision-making skills) appropriate to their age and developmental stage. Achievement could

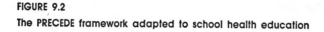

FIGURE 9.2
The PRECEDE framework adapted to school health education

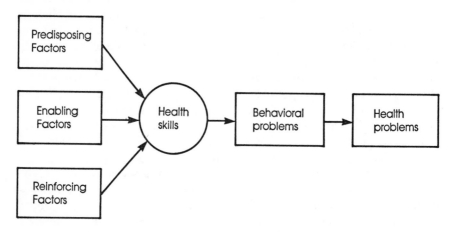

be assessed by means of short descriptions of situations dealing with potential health problems that students would work through after they had completed a unit of study. If a variety of response options were incorporated, students would have opportunities to apply their knowledge and skills in making health choices. Such an approach has dual benefits. One, it allows evaluation of students' ability to *apply* their knowledge, skills, and decision-making powers to a variety of health problems. Two, it has great potential for being an additional source of learning. This kind of evaluation is an integral part of the learning process, an undertaking that actively engages both teachers and students, not something that is "tacked on" to simplify the assignment of grades.

By acknowledging "health skills" objectives, school health educators place themselves in reach of establishing meaningful yet attainable goals. They represent outcomes for which teachers can realistically be held accountable.

The pressures for accountability in school health education are certain to increase. And unless steps are taken to clarify the specific immediate purpose of school health education, programs may be judged on criteria that are inappropriate and unrealistic given the state of the art and the state of organization and support for school education. PRECEDE is a context in which these steps may be productively taken.

Some readers may be concerned about the "problem" focus of the PRECEDE framework. It may appear that PRECEDE reduces school health education to a narrow "disease" orientation or medical model, both antithetical to such current trends as "self-awareness," "holistic health," "wellness" and "positive health." The rationale for our focusing on social and health problems has already been well established. The problem focus notwithstanding, the overriding commitment health education planners make when electing to use PRECEDE is to *specificity*. They commit themselves to dealing not only with specific problems, but with specific objectives, specific behaviors, and, consequently, with specific health education as well. Orderly and specific planning is a prerequisite to reliable evaluation of school health education both in terms of intermediate health skills and in terms of longer-range outcomes.

SUMMARY

In this chapter we test the applicability of the PRECEDE framework to school health education. A review of the history and current status of health education in schools reveals a vigorous field in which innovation and diversity in the classroom have been the rule, but without a clear relationship to the community, without a systematic process of setting priorities for health or behavioral problems, and without a firm grounding in scientific evidence linking the educational activities to the impact or outcomes for which educators will be held accountable. Evaluation has been the exception rather than the rule.

When the PRECEDE framework for planning is applied to school health education, the value of starting the process of curriculum development with diagnosis of the community is demonstrated. Establishing a clear relationship between health education in the schools and the quality of life and health concerns of the community, with community representatives consulted in the planning process, achieves a recognition and support for the value of school health education that is historically lacking.

The controversial question of whether behavior should be an expected goal in school health education is analyzed. Applying the PRECEDE framework, we argue that health behavior and the development or adaptation of behavior are inescapable goals if school health education is expected to have any influence on health or quality of life. Where the PRECEDE framework requires elaboration to accommodate the circumstances of school health education is in the more immediate impact that health education could be expected to have on knowledge and skills. We identify three levels at which evaluation can strengthen health education in the "poverty cycle" of performance, impact, benefits, and support. At the level of impact evaluation we suggest that communities should reasonably be able to hold school health educators accountable for assuring that children at the end of a given school year will be able to make the health-related decisions they will face in the coming year.

This criterion suggests approaches to measuring and evaluating health knowledge and skills, including decision-making skills. The goals of knowledge and skills are both attainable and measurable. They are also relevant to health if they have been clearly derived from epidemiological and behavioral diagnoses of the community and the age ranges for which the curriculum is being planned.

EXERCISES

1.   For a specific grade level, describe a procedure for determining the social and health concerns and needs of the community related to children at the next age. For example, if you are going to plan a health education curriculum for grade five, how will you determine the concerns and needs of parents and others in the community pertaining to the quality of life and health problems of children in the ten- to eleven-year age range?

2.   Specify the behaviors and the skills necessary to enable children at that age to manage effectively the threats, challenges, or opportunities related to an important health problem that might be identified in the epidemiological diagnosis of exercise 1.

3.   Write a description of a situation that would be typical of the circumstances in which a child of this age would have to make a decision concerning action that might influence his or her health. Your scenario should be a realistic case example of a decision-making situation that would call on the knowledge or skill developed in the curriculum for this grade level, and it should ask the child who would read your scenario to identify or select a course of action such as seeking more information, resisting peer pressure, or purchasing one food in preference to another.

10

Applications of PRECEDE to Patient Care

HEALTH EDUCATION has been an important aspect of patient care since the evolution of nursing practice from the Nightingale model of helping the helpless[1] to the primary focus of nursing today on behavior: "The phenomena with which nurses are concerned are [individuals'] health-seeking and coping behaviors as [they strive] to attain health."[2] Health education is vital to clinical practice. And the relationship is reciprocal. Nurses and other patient-care providers represent an extraordinary potential for expanding health education activities in all realms of health care. Nurses, physicians, dentists, and dietitians work with patients and their families in all stages of health and illness in a variety of health-care settings, including hospitals, private offices, industry, rural counties and inner-city neighborhoods. Nurses represent the largest single category of health workers (906,000 active nurses in 1975);[3] but what is said in this chapter concerning nurses can apply almost equally to other clinicians and providers including physicians, dentists, dietitians, pharmacists and others, though in smaller numbers and different ways.

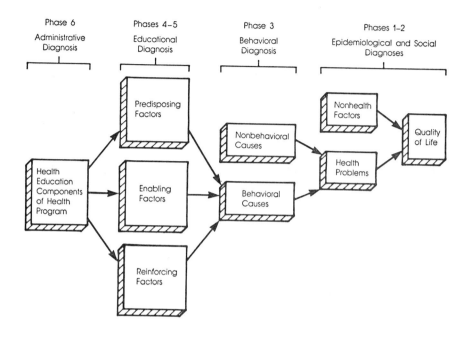

Phase 6
Administrative
Diagnosis

Phases 4–5
Educational
Diagnosis

Phase 3
Behavioral
Diagnosis

Phases 1–2
Epidemiological and Social
Diagnoses

Health Education Components of Health Program

Predisposing Factors

Enabling Factors

Reinforcing Factors

Nonbehavioral Causes

Behavioral Causes

Nonhealth Factors

Health Problems

Quality of Life

Despite the factors supporting and encouraging their involvement in health education, nurses have had difficulty finding time for educational activities.[4] The usual constraints of other duties, limited money, and insufficient personnel resources, coupled with inadequate preparation of nurses for health education, reduce both the quantity and quality of these activities. A 1977 survey of 390 nurses from hospitals and public health agencies revealed both their interest and their problems in incorporating education into practice. Although public health nurses devoted three times more hours per week to education than did hospital nurses (15.1 hours versus 4.4), both groups placed high priority on that aspect of nursing care. Two-thirds of the public health nurses were satisfied with the time they alloted to education; only 40 percent of the hospital nurses were so satisfied. Barriers cited by the hospital nurses included work shifts (night hours are not always conducive to teaching; rotating shifts disrupt teaching efforts), lack of time, and turnover of personnel.[5]

161

An additional barrier is that a major proportion of nurses and other patient-care providers work in acute-care facilities where physical-care needs predominate. With patients experiencing acute or grave illnesses, almost invariably physical care will have priority in patient-care plans. Maintaining physical integrity and assuring safe, prompt implementation of highly technical treatments are cardinal. Understandably, teaching and guidance must wait for life-threatening crises to pass. As the needs of patients become less determined by acute illness, however, increasing time, emphasis, and effort can be given to educational needs. Chronic illness, rehabilitation, pregnancy, childhood development, and aging are examples of situations in which educational needs become salient.

THE NURSING PROCESS AS A MODEL OF PATIENT CARE

The medical model of patient care and the nursing process both are problem-solving processes directed toward clinical problems. Like PRECEDE, both require data collection, problem identification, planning, implementation, and evaluation. The nursing process, however, focuses more than the medical model on positive health behaviors, family strengths and weaknesses, and potential for growth and self-care. As part of their socialization into the nursing process, nurses learn how to gather complete information on an individual as a member of a family, community, and cultural group and how to plan care around the unique qualities and particular needs of that individual. In planning care nurses are expected to distinguish between needs with high and low priorities as well as to determine which interventions (physical care, education, counseling, support, referral, etc.) are most appropriate. After reaching agreement with patients on goals and care plans, nurses, in collaboration with co-workers and the patients and their families, implement interventions and continually monitor their success.

The similarities between the nursing process and the phases of the PRE-CEDE framework are obvious. Both are step-by-step, problem-solving models based on assessment, planning, implementation, and evaluation. The planner is expected to identify and rate problems according to their importance and to the necessity for giving them immediate attention. The patient, client, or community is expected to participate in the planning process. Continual feedback and readjustment are expected in both models. And both assume reliance on scientific and valid data to the extent possible.

What are the differences in the two models? They are mainly differences of emphasis. In the nursing process, the nurse assesses the problems of an individual and plans care for that individual. In the PRECEDE framework a population or aggregate rather than an individual is the basic unit for planning. PRE-CEDE requires epidemiologic, social-survey, and demographic data for the identification of prominent social and health problems in a group under study and for narrowing those problems to the one or two that are important enough to the population to be target(s) of the program. Often there is a political dimension to health education planning that is absent from the nursing process. In addition, PRECEDE deals specifically and primarily with educational needs; whereas the nursing process may focus variably on physical, emotional, or educational needs (an aspect of the nursing process that we shall discuss in more detail later).

These differences suggest the usefulness of the PRECEDE framework to patient-care practice according to three distinct perspectives. The first perspective is community health care, where the planning process is most like the PRECEDE planning approach because both are oriented toward total community needs. The second perspective is administrative. Administrators or staff apply the PRECEDE framework to the planning that they do for organizations or groups such as clinics, voluntary agencies, and inpatient units. The final perspective is that of individual practitioners working with individual patients. How can the PRECEDE framework be applied there?

COMMUNITY HEALTH NURSING AS A MODEL OF COMMUNITY HEALTH CARE

The PRECEDE framework, in taking problems determined to be of greatest importance to a population as bases for programs, is similar to other needs-assessment paradigms in community health nursing. Nurses are expected to survey the social and health needs of an entire area, using demographic and epidemiologic information, and to set areawide priorities. Program planning then proceeds in terms of those priorities, with interventions potentially coming at all levels—political, institutional, agency, family, group, and individual.[6] Such a planning approach is described in useful detail by Reinhardt and Chatlin, who stress broad consideration of social and health needs of communities and use by nurses of new planning methodologies.[7]

Public health nurses need make only one adjustment, then, to use the PRECEDE framework. They must add behavioral and educational diagnoses to their traditional planning process. When nurses (and colleagues) are called on to develop programs in which education is just one of many components, they will have to complement the PRECEDE framework by planning for the noneducational interventions to be directed at nonbehavioral

FIGURE 10.1
Integrating PRECEDE with patient care

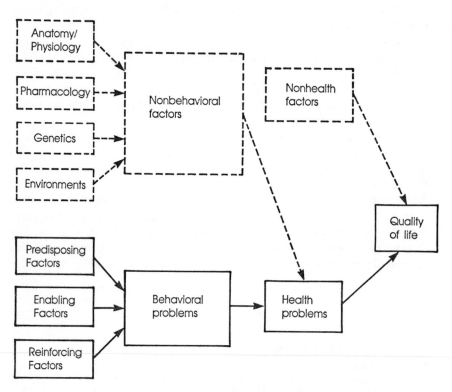

factors influencing health, as shown in figure 10.1. This should not be difficult because PRECEDE dovetails neatly with the nursing process and other
sound planning approaches. As we have emphasized, failure to define objectives precisely and to develop appropriate evaluation procedures has im-
paired the effectiveness of all health education programs. Community health
nurses, as other health educators, can find in the PRECEDE planning framework a quickly incorporated method that overcomes weaknesses currently
evident in community health programs.

The clinician must give as much attention to the nonbehavioral factors
determining health outcomes as to the behavioral. For every predisposing educational factor the physician or nurse must give equal attention to a predisposing genetic or physiological factor such as blood pressure, weight, or previous medical history. For every effort to enable behavioral adjustments the
pharmacist or nurse must attend to enabling physiological adjustments by

monitoring the pharmacological factors such as the dosage and administration of prescribed pills or insulin injections. For every attempt to reinforce patient behavior through education of family members, the dietician or nurse must give comparable attention to the environmental factors in the hospital, home, or work place that will reinforce health improvements independent of behaviors, such as adequate shelter, warmth, facilities, and food.

Each health professional who provides direct patient care must be concerned with a variety of biological and physical determinants of health, but increasingly with the changing character of health problems presented for care, clinicians must have a similar concern with behavioral determinants.

PLANNING FOR GROUPS

There are numerous occasions in patient care when it is appropriate to develop programs on the basis of the needs of a group rather than according to individuals' needs. For example, a medical director or director of nursing for a hospital, a chief nurse or chief resident in a comprehensive child-care clinic, a head nurse on an oncology unit, a family nurse practitioner, a hospital pharmacist or dietitian, a staff nurse in a maternity clinic—all might wish to set priorities for the total population under their care. PRECEDE offers a new approach to achieving that goal. The usual approach consists of a clinician's dealing with each patient and family as they present themselves for care. Each is assessed for most pressing needs and for strengths and weaknesses. Care plans are then prepared with attention to the full gamut of health needs, the importance of the various needs to the patient, and the probability that medical or nursing interventions will achieve the desired outcomes. Seldom do nurses or other clinicians survey the needs in an entire case load to identify particularly pressing or dangerous problems (or potential problems) before planning how they will distribute their time and effort.

Looking at a maternity clinic as an example, a nurse might review all patients' records and conduct a small survey in an attempt to identify the most prevalent problems within that population. Suppose two overriding problems were identified: iron deficiency anemia and a high incidence of prematurity. The nurse could identify patients who were at greatest risk to develop those problems (based on known correlates such as age, socioeconomic status, nutritional status, history of premature infants, etc.) and plan special interventions for that high-risk subgroup. Although the interventions would likely involve medical treatment and care, education would surely be an essential component. Using the PRECEDE framework, the nurse would identify the behaviors that contributed to iron deficiency anemia and prematurity (health problems) and then tease out the predisposing, enabling, and reinforcing factors contributing to the behavior. In the case of iron deficiency anemia, *diet* is too general a statement to be useful in changing a health behavior. More specific goals such as *eating foods that are high in iron or iron-enriched* or *taking iron medication as prescribed* would be appropriate statements of health behaviors that an educational program might increase.

Once the specific behaviors were identified and concrete objectives set for each behavior, the nurse could then determine general patterns pertaining to the causal factors. Predisposing factors could be explored by means of such questions as: What do the patients *know* about iron deficiency anemia? Do they *believe* they have a problem? Do they have *cultural* eating *habits*? Do they *believe* dieting *changes* or medication *will help*? Enabling factors are addressed by such questions as: Do patients have the *skills* necessary to modify their behavior? Are medications and appropriate foods *accessible*? Finally, reinforcing factors are considered: Do patients have *family and peer support* for dieting changes? Are other *health-care professionals willing to reinforce* behavioral changes? Such specificity gives greater visibility to the educational endeavor, facilitates linking the various interventions of the program into a coherent whole, helps the patients participating in the program measure their progress (or lack thereof), and helps the nurse know when behaviors and high-risk statuses change, and, ultimately, when a health problem is coming under control.

Considering the needs of an entire group under care makes it possible to identify and ameliorate problems that might otherwise have a negative effect on a large percentage of the group. That it is possible to discern important problems and develop programs to deal with them reinforces the validity of groups as targets for educational interventions. Offering group experiences to patients and families who share a problem not only is a more efficient use of resources but also may be more effective for patient learning.[8]

WORKING WITH INDIVIDUAL PATIENTS

Turning now to how clinicians might incorporate the PRECEDE framework into planning of care for individual patients, it might be advantageous to review the nursing process briefly. The process consists of assessment, planning, implementation, and evaluation. It focuses on the physical, emotional, and social well-being of the patient and is ongoing in that the progress of the client is closely scrutinized, goals are constantly being readjusted, and new or adapted interventions planned.

One way to see more specifically the commonalities between the PRE-CEDE framework and the nursing process is to analyze the PRECEDE model in each of its phases. PRECEDE calls first for looking at social problems that affect quality of life and hypothesizing about the relationship of those problems to prominent health problems. The approach in nursing to assessing individuals is quite similar, although stated in different terms. Nurses are expected to analyze an individual's total functioning, including the extent to which major role obligations (as wife, student, worker, father, etc.) are being met. Problems related to major family dysfunction are to be given greatest priority.[9] For example, an illness that keeps the breadwinner from working takes priority over illnesses interfering with social activities (unless the individual is an adolescent, for instance, for whom social acceptance is critical in terms of development). Social factors and quality of life, then, do figure prominently in nursing assessments of individuals and families.

At the next phase of the PRECEDE framework, health problems are differentiated from nonhealth problems. The point of this is to make sure that the health care will be directed toward appropriate targets and that the health worker will understand the impact of *other* problems on quality of life. Nurses dealing with families often must distinguish between health and nonhealth problems and occasionally must guide families in dealing with nonhealth problems. Referral to a wide range of social and community resources is common.

Perhaps the major difference between the two procedures is evident in phase 3 of PRECEDE, when the health education planner begins to deal more exclusively with behavioral problems, while nurses often must devote a greater deal of time and energy to the nonbehavioral, biological determinants of health problems. This is true for nursing not only in hospital and ambulatory settings but also in industry, community, and school settings. If one were to depict this responsibility in terms of the PRECEDE framework, it might look as shown in figure 10.1.

Given this expanded perspective, a nurse's general data base on a health problem will extend well beyond the requirements set forth in the PRECEDE framework. A nurse will want to see the behavioral and nonbehavioral components as distinct but interrelated. This point of view should at the same time that it fosters attention to educational needs encourage an integrated response to a patient's total needs. The interplay of behavioral and nonbehavioral factors might be seen in a case in which a nurse works with an adult male to improve his control of high blood pressure. The nurse would carry out an educational diagnosis, for instance, around the patient's failure to take medication regularly, a behavioral problem. In meeting with the patient, however, he or she, besides being interested in whether the patient was following the therapy plan, would be observing the patient for signs of untoward reaction to the medication and checking for complications of any accompanying physical problem such as cardiac disease or diabetes. Monitoring the patient's physical status and his reactions to the medications, counseling for depression he may be feeling because of a perceived limited work future, and referring him to an ophthalmologist for a needed eye examination are examples of noneducational interventions the nurse may need to interweave with the teaching plan. Such additional concerns are common for the clinician and are not addressed in the PRECEDE model.

In the next phase of the PRECEDE framework, the planner is asked to identify the predisposing, enabling, and reinforcing factors contributing to the behavioral problem. Nurses have always included such information in their histories,[10] but in different, more general ways, PRECEDE contributes a structure for organizing the data and for planning interventions, suggesting how the general information can be gathered and organized around a specific health problem and a specific health behavior. Using PRECEDE encourages clinicians to identify one or two health problems of particular importance, to select relevant behaviors affecting the problem, and then to gather patient information relevant to the behavior in such a way that priorities for change become clear. The data base will reveal the predisposing, enabling, and reinforcing factors impinging on the behaviors that the clinician and patient have chosen to work on. The problem-oriented approach to record keeping, which is gaining popularity in patient care, lends itself to the problem-specific assessment and planning recommended in the PRECEDE framework. Clinicians using problem-oriented records may find it easier to gather and record data around individual problems.

After the major factors contributing to the negative behavior have been ascertained, it is possible to plan the educational interventions. What will be needed is a sensitive balancing of educational and other objectives. One positive outcome of clearly focusing on educational needs is that it helps the practitioner deal with conflicting pressures on his or her time and energy. As reflected in figure 10.1, clinicians must respond to nonbehavioral needs of patients, especially in acute-care settings, in which the one-on-one clinical approach predominates. In those settings educational programs often are not granted very much organizational support, and nurses may find their priorities superseded by those of other providers or of the agency. By using the PRECEDE framework nurses can counteract at least some of the pressures by skillfully reducing the teaching aims to a limited number of behaviors and factors. Having clear-cut objectives will help target interventions; it can also make the teaching efforts more visible and acceptable.

WHY IT MAKES SENSE TO APPLY PRECEDE TO PATIENT CARE

We have identified seven reasons why the PRECEDE framework is especially useful in promoting health education in patient care.

1. *Planned* programs, based on documented needs, are more likely to win support from key personnel such as administrators and physicians. Administrators are able to see why certain problems are given priority over others; outcomes are spelled out; and potential benefits to the agency are made more evident. Similarly, physicians and other co-workers can see how educational interventions dovetail with other types of interventions (medications, surgery, physical therapy, diet, etc.). It is often not possible to garner support and cooperation by speaking in general terms of "changing behavior" or "teaching." The PRECEDE framework facilitates clear enunciation of high-priority health problems, health behaviors, and desired changes. When outcomes are clearly stated, they are often found to relate directly to medical regimens (e.g., improved compliance, weight reductions, appointment keeping), a phenomenon that encourages cooperation.

2. PRECEDE focuses on populations or groups, an emphasis greatly needed in medicine and nursing practice, where the one-on-one clinical approach has predominated.[11] Nursing (because of its limited resources) and medicine (because of its dwindling resources relative to costs) must be disciplined in allocating their resources. PRECEDE provides a mechanism for assessing an aggregate (whether an inpatient unit, an outpatient clinic, an industry, a day-care center, or an entire city), choosing key problems and behaviors, and setting specific objectives as outcomes of the educational interventions.

3. In a similar manner, the PRECEDE framework supports the clinical practitioner in identifying subgroups of a population under care who for medical, social, or economic reasons are at high risk for getting ill or not recovering. If nurses or physicians know which patients or groups have the highest concentration of negative predisposing, enabling, and reinforcing factors, they know which have the greatest need of educational interventions.

4. One aspect of the PRECEDE framework that has received little attention is the fact that enabling and reinforcing factors relate specifically to the providers and the health-care system and to the impact of these on patient behavior. Nurses and social workers have long recognized and contended with the burdens that patients and families

shoulder because they are dealing with the health-care system. PRE-CEDE acknowledges the interaction of patients and the health-care system in both its positive and negative manifestations by calling for identification of the patient's perceptions of how these factors affect specific health behaviors and problems. If clinicians find that previous negative experiences are deterring patients from adopting positive behaviors, they (and others involved in the program planning) can intervene in ways designed to eliminate or minimize the negative reinforcing factors.[12]

5. Participation of the patient or community in identifying and mobilizing around its problems is an important element of PRECEDE. Such participation has always been important to nursing. A client is expected to play a major role in determining his or her own health plans, whether that client is a patient with newly diagnosed diabetes, a family dealing with an emotionally disturbed child, a neighborhood striving to eradicate rats, or a youth group involved in recreation projects.[13]

6. Of particular interest to clinicians is the assistance the PRECEDE framework can provide in developing educational plans that cut across agency boundaries. Take, for example, a program developed for pregnant adolescents. Nurses and other providers will be working with these girls during the prenatal, labor, delivery, and postpartum phases of pregnancy in their homes, prenatal clinics, several hospital units, and in postpartum and well-baby clinics. An integrated educational plan will help practitioners in each of these settings make contributions appropriate to the previously identified learning needs and to the previously determined contributions of others involved throughout the maternity cycle. Such a coordinated approach, promoting agreed-on goals, fosters efficient use of resources and can have a great impact.

7. All disciplines have a need to document the results of their efforts. With its emphasis on evaluation, the PRECEDE framework offers an array of avenues for investigation. Such research not only will confirm or deny the usefulness of specific programs or activities but also will generate new hypotheses for subsequent study.

SUMMARY

This chapter shows some of the similarities between the nursing process as a model of patient care and the principles of PRECEDE. The medical model of patient care has some similarities but does not place as much emphasis on health, patient participation in setting objectives for care, behavior, and self-care as do the nursing process and PRECEDE.

The PRECEDE planning framework is valuable to patient care because it stresses: (1) the selection of health problems based on epidemiologic and other data, thereby encouraging efficient use of resources for vulnerable groups and problems; (2) the logical ordering of data to understand components of the health problem and to plan appropriate interventions; (3) the formal preparation of program and learning objectives that lend themselves to evaluation; and (4) the collaboration of both clients and providers.

In this chapter we illustrate how the PRECEDE framework can be used by clinicians in their work with individual patients. The framework gives visibility to the educational needs of patients and can help promote formal planning of programs to meet those needs. Through systematic incorporation of the planning processes inherent in the use of PRECEDE, providers of direct patient care will sharpen their effectiveness in helping others cope productively with the real and potential health threats confronting them. They will also be led to address health in a broad community context.

Throughout this book we urge just such a broadening of perspective on health problems for those whose work in health is confined to clinical, classroom, or occupational settings. We stress the need for specificity in defining and targeting health education priorities as well. Both outlooks are necessary if the context and the reach of health education are to be expanded while the spread of scarce educational resources is limited to those problems and targets where they can do the most good.

EXERCISES

1. For a given clinical setting, describe the distribution of health problems presented by patients and justify the selection of a particular problem as the first priority for health education planning.

2. For the priority health problem, show the procedures you would follow in conducting a behavioral diagnosis and write a behavioral objective for the highest-priority behavior to be addressed in this population of patients.

3. For the chosen behavior, develop an inventory of predisposing, enabling, and reinforcing factors, set priorities on one or two of each, and write educational objectives for these.

APPENDIX A
A Community Demonstration Project: Education and Communication for Local Health Services

A $3,500 GRANT was awarded to the Health Education Center, Maryland State Department of Health and Mental Hygiene, during 1975 and 1976 for the purpose of developing "Education and Communication for Local Health Services," a project designed to broaden the perception and understanding of county residents regarding local health department services. The project was to be conducted in a single county, and a guidebook as well as generic informational materials were to be developed and made available to other jurisdictions in the state.

Adapted from Katherine McCarter, Sharon Dorfman, and Carolyn Hochreiter, *Health Education Strategies for Local Health Departments,* with permission of the Health Education Center, Maryland State Department of Health and Mental Hygiene, Baltimore, 1976.

173

Meetings were held with the health officers and staffs of four counties to determine where the project could best be implemented. Although all counties had needs and interests appropriate to the project, Washington County was chosen as the site of the demonstration effort. The reasons for the choice included staff readiness, health officer commitment, geographic area currently unserved by the local health department, and availability of a local staff person (health educator) to work with the project staff as a major assignment and to ensure ongoing follow-through.

On the basis of meetings with the health officer and key health department staff members, it was determined that a project would be developed to gain local support for the establishment of a permanent location in southern Washington County from which health department services could be delivered.

The need for increased services in southern Washington County was strongly felt by the health department staff and was expressed in the county's five-year plan. Baseline data about this part of the county was obtained from existing reports and studies from public and private planning and service agencies.

SOUTHERN WASHINGTON COUNTY – BASELINE DATA

Bounded on the west by the Potomac River and on the east by the Frederick County line, southern Washington County is a rural area encompassing five election districts. The lower half of the area is divided by a mountain range that runs from the extreme southern tip of the county north to the town of Keedysville. This mountain range divides the lower half into eastern and western portions and creates a barrier to communications and transportation between the two sections.

Most of the population of southern Washington County resides in the northern half of the area near the incorporated towns of Sharpsburg, Keedsville, and Boonsboro. This area has an unusually large percentage (26 percent) of people with incomes below poverty level. The election districts in Keedysville and Rohrersville have a high percentage of elderly residents (Keedysville, 11 percent; Rohrersville, 14 percent). Substandard housing is an important health-related factor in the area. According to the 1970 Census, of the 1,078 substandard dwelling units in the area, 893 were occupied. This number represents 31 percent of all housing units occupied in the five election districts. Nearly one out of three families is living in housing without central heating or a complete plumbing system.

The 9,600 residents of the target area have very few health services available to them without traveling considerable distance. There is one physician practicing full-time in Boonsboro and a physician who practices half-time in Sharpsburg. A psychiatrist has recently moved his residence to the small town of Brownsville but practices primarily in the Washington, D.C., area. Thus the ratio of primary-care physicians to population in the target area is 1:6,400. This is a dramatically lower ratio than for the county as a whole (1:1,932) or the state (1:1,497). In fact, five more primary-care physicians would be necessary to match the area to the current state level.

Depending on the part of the area in which they live, the residents travel to Hagerstown, and Frederick County, Maryland, or nearby West Virginia to get medical services.

Two dentists have a full-time joint practice in Boonsboro. There are no other dentists practicing in the target area. Since the closing of the commercial pharmacy in Boonsboro several years ago, there have been no pharmacy services available in the area.

There are two long-term care institutions in the target area, both located near Boonsboro. A church-supported nursing home has 135 beds. The Reeder Memorial Home, a multilevel health facility, has 146 beds. Washington County Hospital in Hagerstown is the main inpatient acute-care facility serving the county, but some residents in the southern area go to the Frederick County Hospital or the hospital in Charles Town, West Virginia.

The Department of Health, Education, and Welfare has identified the Keedysville and Rohrersville election districts as being medically underserved because of the lack of physicians, the high percentage of elderly among the population, and the high percentage of indigent residents.

LOCAL HEALTH DEPARTMENT SERVICES

The Washington County Health Department provides home health and public health nursing visits to residents of southern Washington County. However, both types of services are underused because there are few physicians to order them and because the health department, lacking permanent headquarters in the area, is not visible to the southern county residents.

The health department holds monthly itinerant clinics to deliver well-child services in Sharpsburg and Brownsville. Both these clinics are held in church buildings, and equipment must be transported each time a clinic is held.

Water and waste water installation inspections and other environmental health services are provided as requested or on a scheduled basis in the area.

Area residents requiring health department services for family planning, maternity care, tuberculosis, venereal disease, mental health, addictions, and specialty clinics for children must travel from twenty-five to forty-five minutes to the department's central headquarters.

THE EDUCATIONAL DIAGNOSIS

On the basis of the baseline data available, an educational diagnosis was developed. The framework for this diagnosis was PRECEDE. Information to assess the enabling factors was readily available at the start of the project, but it was necessary to design methods to obtain data concerning predisposing and reinforcing factors. Highlights of the educational diagnosis are presented below.

```
┌──────────────────────┐
│                      │
│    Social problem    │
│                      │
└──────────────────────┘
```

The following are indicators of social problems or quality-of-life concerns:

1. Of the residents of the five election districts in southern Washington County, 26.1 percent have incomes below the poverty level.
2. Substandard housing units make up 31.3 percent of the total.
3. The lower half of the area is divided by a mountain range, which creates a barrier to communications and transportation.

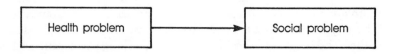

Health problems are indicated by:

1. high infant-mortality rate
2. low physician-patient ratio
3. absence of adequate community water and sewerage systems
4. inaccessible private and public health services

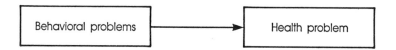

Behavioral problems exist with both consumers and providers of health services. These are:

1. Consumers
    a) underuse of existing limited health services
    b) lack of adherence to the best possible health practices regarding preventive actions and compliance with prescribed regimens
2. Providers, Washington County Health Department—County health department has not been able to respond to the health services needs of the target area fully and effectively

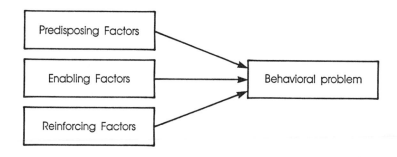

Predisposing Factors
(demographic variables, knowledge, attitudes, values, and norms)

1. Consumers—Information about predisposing factors of the target area was not available. A community health survey was designed and conducted to assess predisposing factors such as:
    a) knowledge, attitudes, and beliefs about personal health and individual responsibility for health
    b) effects of prior health-care experiences
    c) knowledge, attitudes, and beliefs regarding the health-care system in general and the county health department specifically
2. Providers, Washington County Health Department—A staff survey was conducted to determine:
    a) staff knowledge, attitudes, and beliefs regarding health needs and interests of the target area gained through study of available data and contact with patients

b) knowledge, attitudes, and beliefs regarding staff role and responsibility in the community

Enabling Factors
(availability of resources, accessibility, and referrals)

1. Consumers—Initial baseline data identified:
   a) the scarcity of physicians, pharmacists, and other medical personnel in the area
   b) financial considerations and distance to needed services
   c) limitations of county health department services to this area
2. Providers, Washington County Health Department—Information about the county health department indicated:
   a) resources were insufficient to acquire space for delivery of expanded services
   b) staff assigned to the area commuted from twenty-five to forty-five minutes from offices in Hagerstown
   c) distance and resource constraints did not allow visibility or close communications with the community
   d) philosophy and resources precluded the provision of primary care to the target area

Reinforcing Factors
(attitudes and actions of health personnel, family, and others)

1. Consumers—Information about reinforcing factors was not available. The community health survey was needed to provide information about:
   a) consumer perception of personal health status
   b) quality of interaction with health professionals
2. Providers, Washington County Health Department—
   The negative reinforcing factors were:
   a) previous attempts to establish a base of operations for providing health department services had not been successful
   b) local efforts to recruit a pharmacist to establish a drugstore had failed
   c) the staff felt that the target-area residents did not know about existing health department services or the health department's role as a catalyst in developing an adequate health service delivery system

A positive reinforcing factor was: Individual community leaders in the target area expressed to the health department concern about inadequate health services.

The enabling factors identified in the educational diagnosis were so compelling that strategies to influence predisposing and reinforcing factors were not expected to be effective until measures were taken to change the enabling factors. Therefore, change of the enabling factors became the focus of the objectives for the project. Once these objectives could be achieved, knowledge about the consumer predisposing and reinforcing factors gained from the community health survey and from continuing contact with the community would be used in planning and delivering expanded health services.

Educational Objectives

Objective 1: After one year, residents of southern Washington County will provide adequate facilities for delivery of health department services. Adequate facilities are defined as:

    a) office space for four nurses, one sanitarian, and one secretary
    b) clinic space with a waiting room, examination rooms, laboratory, and a conference room

Objective 2: After six months, community volunteers and community organizations will provide support services to health department activities. Support services consist of:

    a) participation in planning for improved health and community services
    b) participation on a facility search committee
    c) involvement in the development, implementation, and evaluation of a community health survey
    d) collection of additional baseline data
    e) offers of volunteer services

Objective 3: By the end of one year, five organizations in southern Washington County will initiate and carry out health education-related activities. Health education-related activities are:

    a) education of membership about health-service needs of the area
    b) education of legislators, county commissioners, and other county leaders about health-service needs

Objective 4: By the end of one year, residents of the target area will express their demand for needed health services in terms of:

a) vocal demands at community meetings
b) findings of the community health survey
c) media coverage of project and recognition of health needs
d) participation in efforts to improve health care (objectives 1 and 2)
e) greater use of new facility than of Hagerstown clinic facilities

Objective 5: After one year, the Washington County Health Department will take steps to expand or reorganize its services to the citizenry according to confirmed community health-care needs and available health department resources. "Taking steps to expand or reorganize" consists of:

a) establishing clinic services based in southern Washington County
b) establishing a permanent base of operations for staff
c) assuming a leadership role in the demonstration project and its implementation
d) collecting baseline data
e) participating in the community health survey
f) making staff time available for project implementation
g) changing clinic services offered or hours and days offered

Community health-care needs are confirmed by:

a) baseline data
b) findings of the community health survey
c) findings of the staff survey

Objective 6: After one year, the community will use existing health department services more appropriately; appropriateness will be determined according to criteria established in consultations with various health personnel.

EDUCATIONAL STRATEGIES

Since the objectives focused on enabling factors, the educational strategies emphasized community-organization techniques. Implicit in the decision to use community-organization strategies and in the concept of a demonstration project was the understanding that active participation and commitment of the Washington County Health Department staff would be essential.

Throughout the implementation of the demonstration project, conscious effort was made to seek the active involvement of members of the health department staff, especially those assigned to and directly involved in the delivery of services in the target area. A staff steering committee was formed and involved throughout the project in:

1. general data collection
2. contribution to understanding of the target area by sharing of perceptions and knowledge
3. identification of community leaders in target area
4. development of a community health survey
5. formal and informal communications and contacts with significant community leaders

The effectiveness of this strategy was apparent at the end of the demonstration period when the county health department, in concert with the community leadership, was preparing to establish and operate a new health and community services center.

In addition to the staff involvement, a major element in the community-organization strategy was the organization of a community steering committee. This group was formed to identify priority health-service needs and to plan and implement solutions to meet these needs. The decision to establish a local group that would assume leadership for the project was made with a full knowledge of the inherent advantages and disadvantages of this approach. It is a time-consuming process that requires belief in the ability of informed citizens to make appropriate decisions about their health needs. Further, it requires project staff to be flexible in their approach to the project and responsive to the variety of expectations of the community.

The benefits of the community-organization strategy, however, outweighed the disadvantages. Sporadic attempts to increase health resources by health department staff and concerned individuals in the target area had not succeeded in the past. Although an active interest remained on the part of a few, there was no interorganizational structure representative of the total target area that could serve as a forum for joining forces to work on solutions to the problem. By establishing a representative community steering committee, local knowledge of the area's leadership-communications networks and power structures was pooled and directed toward setting objectives and achieving results. Participation in this process provided a continuous learning experience for community participants, health department staff, and project directors.

In addition to the community-organization strategies, communications strategies were employed on a one-to-one, small-group, and areawide basis. The local weekly newspapers covered the progress of the project and the deliberations of the community meetings.

CHRONOLOGY

The major steps in development of the project are outlined according to approximate time frames.

1. March–April 1975—Project directors met with selected county health officers and staff to determine interest and feasibility in conducting a demonstration health education project. Washington County was selected for the project site.
2. May 1975—The staff of the Health Education Center collected initial baseline data and met with health department staff to prepare a project proposal. Six objectives were selected for a project in the southern portion of Washington County and were accepted by the health officer.
3. June 1975—The staff of the Health Education Center met with county health department's staff steering committee to survey staff knowledge and attitudes about health needs and services in southern Washington County and to review the specific objectives of the project.
4. June 1975—The search for available baseline data was expanded and work on constructing a community health survey to obtain necessary but nonexisting data was begun. Research in needs assessment and questionnaire construction was instituted in preparation for the community health survey.
5. July 1975—The staff of the Health Education Center met with the staff steering committee to identify southern Washington County community leaders and to plan for a public meeting to be held in the target area. Stated objectives for the meeting were to introduce the project, to stimulate dialogue, and to obtain a commitment from some of the participants to form a community steering committee.
6. July 1975—A public meeting was held in the Keedysville Municipal Building and was attended by invited community leaders, the health officer of Washington County, and the health department's staff steering committee for the purpose of community mobilization and project implementation.
7. July 1975–February 1976—Community health steering committee meetings:
   a) *Committee membership*—Committee membership was expanded from the original volunteers to include others who were identified and invited to participate as specific expertise was needed.
   b) *Committee structure*—Although most of the activities of the committee were confined to the monthly evening meetings of the

core members, specific assignments were carried out between meetings by task groups and individuals. A member of the health department staff served as chairperson until the group made a selection from among the membership. Minutes were recorded and distributed. All meetings were held in the centrally located Keedysville Municipal Building.

  c) *Committee progress*—As is typical of most groups, the goals of the community health steering committee changed as the group developed cohesiveness and sharpened its perceptions of the health problems. Feelings of frustration from lack of immediate solutions and uneven progress were balanced by a sense of real accomplishment as planning proceeded.

At first the group focused on the immediate problem of locating a building from which existing health department services could be delivered. This action was taken as an initial step even though the committee had lengthy discussions about priority health needs that could not be met by such services.

After several task groups had made an exhaustive survey of available existing structures in the target area and found that none was suitable, the committee was forced to realize that it was not possible to start small and expand over time. Confronted with having to consider the construction of a new facility, the committee recognized its need for additional members with special knowledge and saw the possibility of enlarging its definition of needs beyond those that the health department could meet. Continuing discussions identified the need to provide space for other health services such as primary health care and for health-related human services such as day care for children and special services to the aged.

During this time, the committee realized the value of a community health survey in planning for a new facility, made helpful revisions to an early draft questionnaire, and advised about survey design and procedures.

Explorations into funding possibilities for the new facility led to serious study of the requirements for Appalachia Regional Council (ARC) grants for health-care facilities. It was evident that planning and matching money would need to be assured in order to develop and submit a grant proposal. The committee enlisted the support of several key governmental and private community agencies; secured county government approval of the intent of the project; obtained commitments for planning and matching money; and discovered a school building scheduled to be closed that was suitable for renovation into a health and community services center. This groundwork was sufficient for the steering committee to submit its findings and recommendations for a grant proposal to the residents of the target area.

8. February 1976—A well-publicized and attended public meeting was held in Keedysville, Maryland, to discuss the findings and recommendations of the community steering committee. After presentations by committee members and full discussion by participants, there was strong approval to proceed with preparing a grant proposal to meet the March 1, 1976, Appalachia Regional Council deadline.

The report and recommendations developed by the community steering committee and approved by the community were:

Administration and organization

It was recommended that the county commissioners become the applicants for an ARC grant so that an application could be submitted immediately, making the project eligible for current fiscal-year funds. It was also recommended that the county commissioners place operational responsibility of the center in the hands of a governing board of directors.

The first-year funding application would include a request for funds to modernize and renovate the existing Keedysville Elementary School if it became available for the project at the end of the 1976–77 school year. The board of directors, when formed and incorporated, could make arrangements for various service agencies, such as the health department and the department of education, to use parts of the renovated facility to deliver their services.

Services

a) Satellite health department center

    (1) Health department offices would provide space for relocating current health department staff serving this area of the county.

    (2) Health department clinic space would be sufficient to allow for expanded services. Initially, child health and family planning clinics would be the two services offered most frequently. Other clinics, such as mental health, venereal disease, crippled children, and prenatal would be scheduled according to the needs of the area residents.

b) Preschool day-care center—The board of education indicated an interest in operating a preschool day-care program for working parents.

c) Services for the aging—Services would include health, social services, and recreation.

d) Other community services—Space would be made available to other organizations such as the Department of Social Services, Community Action Council, Vocational Rehabilitation, Extension Service, Senior Citizens, and civic clubs, to provide services and to hold meetings.

e) Primary health care—Planning for primary health care (defined as the kind of medical care most people need most of the time) would be initiated with the approval of the funding application to renovate part of the center to be used for this service. A future funding application would be submitted to cover start-up and operational costs for the primary-care service.

f) Transportation—A transportation network would be developed to support all services provided through the center.

9. February 1976—The committee formally appeared before the mayors and town councils of Boonsboro, Keedysville, and Sharpsburg to obtain their support for the proposal. All three bodies indicated unanimous approval. A formal request for the use of the Keedysville school was made through the health department.

10. February 1976—An instrument for assessing residents' attitudes and knowledge of the local health department and health-care needs and practices in the target area was finalized and pretested. The survey was mailed in a random sample to one in every three households in the target area during February 1976. A telephone follow-up for nonrespondents was conducted by trained community volunteers. The results of the survey when compiled and analyzed will be used in the ongoing implementation of the project.

11. March–April 1976—The grant proposal was submitted to ARC in time to be considered for fiscal year 1977 funds. This was possible through the continued coordinated efforts of many individuals and groups.

    A representative board of directors was organized and will become a community based, nonprofit corporation to receive federal funds and operate the center. At the end of the demonstration-project period, the board had begun its deliberations.

12. May 1976—Project directors from the State Health Education Center withdrew from active participation in the demonstration

project. The Washington County Health Department and community members assumed full responsibility for continuing the project.

EVALUATION

A review of the six objectives delineated in the original demonstration-project proposal for Washington County indicated that although the project continues, substantial progress had already been made toward achieving these objectives.

Objective 1: After one year, residents of southern Washington County will provide adequate facilities for delivery of health department services.

The planned Health and Community Services Center will contain adequate health department space as measured by the established indicators.

Objective 2: After six months, community volunteers and community organizations will provide support services to health department activities.

Citizens have given leadership throughout the entire project and have provided support services as defined in the original objectives. Minutes of the community meetings reflect only a small part of the total support and commitment given this project by citizens of the target area, other individuals, and agencies and officials in the county. In addition, the community health survey indicated high respondent interest in a variety of volunteer roles.

Objective 3: By the end of one year, five organizations in southern Washington County will initiate and carry out health education-related activities.

Throughout the demonstration period, organizations such as the Ruritan clubs, Senior Citizens, and the Community Action Council have been involved in efforts to educate their membership, friends, and neighbors about the need for increased health-care services and to elicit input into the planning process. Currently under way is an effort to develop an organized outreach project to be conducted by volunteer groups and designed to offer all groups in the target area an opportunity to be involved in the continuing development of the Health and Community Services Center.

Additionally, the Community Action Council was directly involved in implementing the telephone follow-up to the community health survey.

Objective 4: By the end of one year, residents of the target area will express their demand for needed health services.

The high level of interest in and support for the establishment of a health and community services center in the target area dramatically demonstrated expressed demand. Response to the community health survey indicated a high level of interest in the establishment of a health and community services center, and respondents indicated their priorities for health services. Consistent media coverage of the project activities expressed and reinforced the demand for expanded services. Although it was originally planned to evaluate "expressed demand" through utilization of a new health department delivery site, this was not possible during the demonstration period.

Objective 5: After one year, the Washington County Health Department will take steps to expand or reorganize its services to the citizenry according to confirmed community health-care needs and available health department resources.

The Washington County Health Department had gone far beyond its original commitment to expand services in the target area. It acted as the catalyst in the development of the ARC grant, which addressed health department services and the establishment of primary care and other supporting community services for the area. The health department plans to use the findings of the community health survey to continue its leadership role in planning for all health services in the target area and in adapting its own services to the expressed needs of that population.

Objective 6: After one year, the community will use existing health department services more appropriately; appropriateness will be determined according to criteria established in consultations with various health personnel.

Since health department services were extremely limited and offered on an infrequent basis in the target area, and since major reorganization will occur as the Health and Community Services Center becomes a reality, there was no feasible way to demonstrate this outcome during the demonstration-project period. As a result, no attempt was made to develop a set of quantifiable measures of utilization patterns.

In addition to an evaluation of the demonstration project according to the stated objectives, a process evaluation was planned. A system of compiling all materials relevant to the project was established. This material was useful for monitoring and coordinating ongoing activities as well as for providing an invaluable single-source record of the project.

EPILOGUE

This demonstration project illustrates the advantage of incorporating carefully planned health education strategies as an integral part of public health programming. It is important to emphasize that for any given public health problem an educational diagnosis must be made and strategies must be selected that will affect the factors identified as influencing the problem. Thus, a problem similar to that addressed by the Washington County project undertaken in another locale may require a different set of strategies. The health education concepts embodied in the demonstration project and described in this report have been applied successfully to health programs as diverse as those dealing with solid waste disposal problems and outpatient noncompliance with prescribed regimens.

APPENDIX B
Patient Education Project: A Clinical Application of the PRECEDE Framework

THE PRECEDE FRAMEWORK can be used for sorting out priorities and designing a patient education program. Although this program we are going to describe had a research objective (the evaluation of cause-and-effect relationships), the logic, the process, and the outcomes are applicable to on-going clinical service programs.[1]

In this case, the priority health problem is morbidity, disability, and mortality due to hypertensive disease. We first give reasons for its choice, then comment on the social problems it creates, the quality of life question. The behavioral aspects of the problem and the design and implementation of the educational program are described next. Finally, we discuss the results of the program.

THE PRIORITY HEALTH PROBLEM: MORBIDITY, DISABILITY, AND MORTALITY DUE TO HYPERTENSIVE DISEASE

An initial step in the PRECEDE approach is to identify a priority health problem. The criteria for selection are importance of the problem (prevalence and severity of impact) and the potential the problem has for resolution through educational means.

The Magnitude of the Problem

"Hypertension disease is a serious mass public health problem despite the fact that, at any given time, a majority of persons with it are symptom-free. Hypertension markedly increases the risk of major cardiovascular complications. . . . It is estimated that there are 20 to 25 million hypertensives in the United States."[2] National Health Examination Survey data indicate that in 1960–62 there were about 12,000,000 white American adults aged eighteen to seventy-nine with hypertensive heart disease, definite or suspect and 3,000,000 black American adults in the same age category, totaling 15,000,000.[3] These numbers, which are substantially greater today, represent a huge pool of people (many of them undiagnosed) with markedly increased risk of premature mortality.[4]

Increased premature mortality is by no means the only problem. Data from the Social Security Administration show a sizable amount of disability in the labor force attributable to hypertensive disease.[5] The economic losses to the individuals involved are great, as are the costs to government and society at large. Overall, of the 330,783 worker-disability allowances in 1968, for example, 24 percent were due to diseases of the circulatory system, with arteriosclerotic heart disease at the top of the list for each of the four major sex-race groups. At least one-third of the coronary cases have hypertension as the major contributing cause in the disabling illness. An even higher proportion of the people disabled by stroke have the same major contributing cause.

These data conclusively rank hypertensive disease and its complications at the top of the list as producers of disability for all of the major sex-race groups in the labor force. As expected from the review of other data, this disease and its complications take a disproportionate toll among black Americans, in view of their high prevalence rates of hypertensive heart disease in particular.

The Cost of Untreated Hypertension

In the United States the sequelae of hypertensive disease are estimated to have indirect costs of $1.7 billion. If the indirect costs of one-third of the premature heart attacks and strokes are added ($5.9 billion), the indirect costs are brought up to $7.6 billion. Add the direct costs, estimated by Stamler at $2 billion a year,[6] and the total estimate of the costs of hypertensive disease in 1967 came to $9 billion. Increases in costs due to inflation, particularly in costs for medical care, would make the costs in 1974 (the beginning of this project) astronomical.

The Available Solution to the Health Problem

The available solution to the problem of hypertension at the present time is a prescribed medical regimen that will reduce blood pressure to a level at which much of the accompanying end-organ damage (indicated in the statistics) can be avoided. The desired outcome for this project is control of blood pressure, not cure for the disease. There is presently no cure.

This antihypertensive regimen is based on data from Veterans Administration field trials indicating that effective comprehensive control programs can cut morbidity, disability, and mortality from hypertensive disease by over 50 percent. The data further indicated that if complications are to be avoided, effective therapy should be continued indefinitely without interruption.[7]

In summary, then, hypertension is a prevalent and costly public problem, but once detected, one that can be treated and controlled through antihypertensive medication.

The Behaviors Implicit in the Solution

The major behaviors that are required and that will form the basis for the control activity are *identification* of hypertensives, *treatment* of hypertensives, and continuation of treatment, referred to generally as *compliance with the medical regimen.*

Before discussing the definition and development of the educational program, let us look at the social problems, or quality of life impact, associated with the health problem.

THE QUALITY OF LIFE IMPACT

Health is not an end in itself, but a means toward the attainment of satisfying and productive lives. The costs to society of supporting people disabled through cardiovascular disease and strokes can be estimated as well as the costs of supporting dependents of wage earners who are the victims of these diseases.

Deaths from disease are considered costly to society when they occur prematurely. In the United States, the impact of hypertension in the male worker in his middle years is particularly striking. The relationship of hypertension to this phenomenon is shown in the following quote from Stamler:

> For the most straightforward and crucial index available, i.e., death from all causes, the 10-year rate was 60 percent higher for men with diastolic pressures 95–105 mm Hg, compared to normotensives, and 200 percent higher for those with hypertension in the range of 105 mm Hg and greater. Note also the 60 percent greater mortality rate from all causes even for the men with diastolic pressures of 85–94 mm Hg. [8]

The impact of the major cardiovascular diseases on the life expectancy of white males is demonstrated in table B.1. Despite reductions in deaths from killer diseases such as pneumonia, life expectancy for the middle and older ages is about the same as it was in the 1900s. The situation is only slightly better for black males and for women of both races.

Vast resources are spent on medical care for people in these older age groups with little effect on life expectancy.

TABLE B.1

Expectation of life (years) of white males, by year and age: United States, 1900–70

Age	Year				
	1900	1920	1940	1960	1970
0	52.8	60.3	65.4	67.4	67.7
5	59.9	62.4	64.3	64.4	64.4
20	47.9	49.1	50.1	50.1	50.1
30	39.6	40.8	40.9	40.9	40.9
40	31.2	31.7	31.7	31.7	31.7
50	23.1	23.2	23.2	23.2	23.2

SOURCE: J. S. Stamler et al., "Hypertension. The Problem and the Challenge," *The Hypertension Handbook* (West Point, Pa.: Merck Sharp & Dohme, 1974). Table prepared by E. A. Lew and F. Seltzer from basic data presented by P. A. Jacobson, *Cohort Survival of Generations Since 1840, Milbank Memorial Fund Quarterly* (July 1964) and publications of The National Center for Health Statistics, Department of Health, Education and Welfare.

The economic losses to government and society from disability and morbidity were alluded to earlier. The misery and suffering reflected in these estimates of disability, morbidity, and premature death can only be imagined. It is not difficult to conclude that this problem has a big impact on our society generally and that the control of hypertension would, besides alleviating emotional distress, make resources available for other pressing needs. Figure B.1 summarizes the steps necessary to resolve the problem.

The conclusion that it should be less expensive in the long run to control hypertension than to care for those who become disabled and economically unproductive because of it formed the basis for a national policy decision and program for the control of the disease. Based on national surveys,[9] the following formula was generally accepted in the early 1970s: One-half the hypertensives are undetected; one-half of the known hypertensives are inadequately treated. This formula, shown in figure B.2, clearly reflected a challenge to both health education and the medical care delivery system for the first half of the 1970s.

FIGURE B.1

Logic of the preventive approach to hypertensive diseases

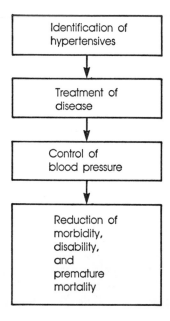

FIGURE B.2

The distribution of awareness (a) and treatment (b) of hypertension:
U.S. population, early 1970s

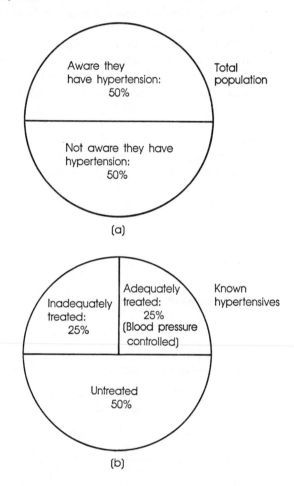

(a)

(b)

THE CONTEXT OF THE PROJECT

In the 1970s the Inter-Society Commission for Heart Disease Resources set
forth in two reports the basic concepts that hypertension is a public health
problem amenable to community efforts in detection, diagnosis, and management and that case finding is essential but of little value unless combined
with referral for care and systematic follow-up.[10] Specific approaches for the

implementation of a national program for primary prevention, detection, and control of hypertension were recommended.

In 1972 the Secretary of the Department of Health, Education, and Welfare established the National High Blood Pressure Education Program as part of the Heart, Lung, and Blood Institute to undertake activities aimed at achieving greater control of blood pressure among hypertensives. The program (authorized under PL 92-423) is specifically designed to increase public and professional awareness of the dangers of high blood pressure, thereby stimulating activities that would result in a decrease in related morbidity and mortality.

In 1974 the National High Blood Pressure Education Research Program, as one of those activities, established a competition for research funds, the research to focus on specific aspects of adherence behavior in hypertension and result in a better understanding of

1. the characteristics of an individual that may relate to adherence behavior
2. the educational interventions that will enhance a patient's initial and long-term adherence to hypertensive therapy

The Health Education Division of Johns Hopkins School of Hygiene and Public Health, along with the Hopkins Health Services Research Center, submitted a proposal to the National Heart, Lung, and Blood Institute as a response to the research opportunity.

PLANNING AND IMPLEMENTATION OF THE PROGRAM

As the beginning of a grant application to carry out research in hypertension patient education, other high blood pressure control programs were reviewed as was the research and practice evidence relating to trends in hypertension screening, referral, diagnosis, and treatment. The logic of an overall strategy for controlling elevated blood pressure was also considered.

The research and practice literature gave little evidence of success in improving blood pressure control in those patients who were under treatment and considerable evidence of an extensive problem that physicians call *noncompliance*. *Noncompliance* refers to the failure of many patients to follow the medical and dietary regimens prescribed by the physicians, which results, in turn, in frequent failure to maintain adequate blood pressure control. Logic indicated that the problem of noncompliance had to be dealt with first. Otherwise, efforts to screen and refer patients into the medical-care system could only result in intensifying the compliance problem. Referral would burden an already overloaded ambulatory-care system with patients who might be even less motivated than those who had come in earlier. There would then be less time per patient, a greater need for standardization of care, and, therefore, less personalized attention to the patient's reasons for noncompliance. [11]

Among the numerous factors associated with inadequate control and noncompliance were inappropriate referrals and lack of physician awareness of such noncompliance. One approach to improving care for hypertensive patients, then, might be an educational program aimed at increasing physician awareness and changing behavior in a manner that would improve referrals, patient education, compliance, and ultimately, control of hypertension.

Providers of care to hypertensive populations vary in their understanding of hypertension and its consequences, and this may influence their diagnosis and their subsequent vigor in pursuing a therapeutic course. Preliminary studies indicated that educational intervention at the provider level might make a significant difference in therapeutic aggressiveness and consequently in the degree of blood pressure control achieved by patients. [12]

Previous studies have documented the probability of patients getting "lost" in the medical-care referral process. The grant application, therefore, also proposed investigation of the adequacy of the referral process for hypertensive patients.

In addition to examining the correlates of the compliance problem in terms of the patients, the providers, and the system to identify where health education efforts might prove most fruitful, the principles and strategies of learning and behavior change were studied. This review led us to conclude that: (1) no single educational intervention could be expected to have a lasting effect on patient behavior unless it was supported by other educational experiences over time; (2) what worked to change the behavior of some patients would not necessarily work for others; and (3) changes in patient behavior were usually associated with changes in certain predisposing, enabling, and reinforcing factors similar to those found to be operating in earlier research on preventive health behavior and health care utilization behavior. [13] The literature on patient education did not provide definitive guidelines on which of the predisposing, enabling and reinforcing factors would be critical in the current problem, but it was clear that all three kinds of factors should be taken into account in planning an educational intervention.

Studies that examined behavioral factors in improving compliance in patients with other diseases were also reviewed. The causal chain that was implied by the conclusions from these reviews was laid out according to the now familiar PRECEDE framework, figure B.3. Note the essential elements of the proposed approach to health education for individuals with hypertension. The program would be directed at three sets of behavioral determinants: predisposing factors, enabling factors, and reinforcing factors. The primary target groups for educational inputs designed to influence these factors were patients themselves in the case of predisposing factors and clinical and supporting staff in the case of enabling and reinforcing factors. Relatives, friends, and other lay individuals and groups are regarded as important channels of communication with patients as sources of reinforcement for behavior.

The Setting

While the literature was being reviewed, the setting in which the proposed project would take place was also under study. From this information the analysis of the enabling factors, as reflected by the impact of the system on the desired outcome, would be derived.

The project was planned for two clinics at the Johns Hopkins Hospital, the general medical clinic and the hypertension clinic. The general medical clinic had an annual volume of 20,000–25,000 scheduled visits. Most patients were black, received Medicaid funds, and lived close to the hospital. Hypertension was the most common principal diagnosis for which visits were made; approximately one-third of the patients were so diagnosed. Of the estimated 4,000 patients treated for hypertension as outpatients at the hospital, 70 percent were seen in the general clinic and the rest in the hypertension clinic. The population at the hypertension clinic, which held morning and afternoon sessions one day a week, was characterized by a higher percentage of males and people aged thirty-nine and under. Few people were over sixty. Further, a greater number of patients in this clinic were in higher income brackets and higher educational brackets.

Numerous discussions and continuous communications took place with hospital staff at all levels to explore the feasibility of the project and the constraints of the clinic settings.

The needs assessment we conducted was more elaborate than one that might be undertaken in a practice setting in which a less rigorous evaluation is required. However, resources and time should be budgeted for some such exploration before initiating any project. Since this allows the project to begin with a firm foundation, the costs are well justified. Projects built on the experience of others and available theory and research are more likely to include precise diagnoses and therefore more likely to be successful.

The proposal, submitted to the National High Blood Pressure Education Research Program, was aimed at the second research objective identified in "Program Announcement and Guidelines" issued for research programs: "better understanding of the educational interventions that will enhance a patient's initial and long-term adherence to hypertensive therapy." The objectives stated in the proposal were as follows:

FIGURE B.3

The first formal application of the PRECEDE framework to hypertension

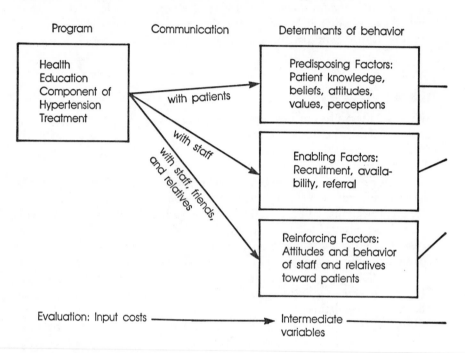

SOURCE: L. W. Green, D. M. Levine, and S. G. Deeds, "Clinical Trials of Health Education for Hypertensive Patients: Design and Baseline Data," **Preventive Medicine** 4 (1975): 417–25.

1. to identify cost-effective and feasible ways to deliver patient care and patient education
2. to identify cost-effective ways to educate professionals and patients to effect behavioral changes that result in the reduction of blood pressure of individuals with hypertension

The proposal, which was funded by National Heart, Lung, and Blood Institute for three years, had the time frame outlined in table B.2, although at the time only the number of interventions were specified, not the content.

The Educational Diagnosis

The project began with surveys and structured conversations with samples of patients and staff. One purpose of these was to establish baseline measures of

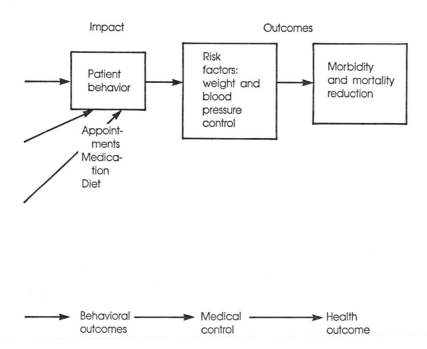

knowledge, attitudes, beliefs, values, perceptions, norms, and behavior. Another was to generate in the staff a degree of involvement and a sense of participation in the planning of the educational programs.

To refine the needs assessment, we weighed the relative importance of the various predisposing, enabling, and reinforcing factors believed to influence compliance behavior and blood pressure. Because of the dearth of standardized instruments or batteries of questions appropriate for measuring the variables, considerable methodological work went into the development and testing of questions and scales on: knowledge of hypertension; blood pressure control; self-reported compliance with medication taking; and the patients' beliefs in the seriousness of hypertension and in the benefits of treating it.[14]

The diagnostic baseline survey had three components: a patient survey, a provider survey, and an examination of the system of care. The patient survey was made on a systematic random sample of 311 clinic patients with essential hypertension treated in the Johns Hopkins Hospital general medical

TABLE B.2
Time plan for the hypertension project

Study funded	May 1974
Baseline study	June–September 1974
Phase I–Clinic interview	March–May 1975
Provider study	March–April 1975
Referral study	July 1975
Phase II—Field interview (family-member study)	July–November 1975
Phase III—Group discussions	January–June 1976
Final field follow-up	June–September 1976
Termination date	April 1977

and hypertension clinics.[15] The provider survey was made of 103 providers in the same clinics.

The examination of the hospital system focused on volume and patterns of referral from clinic to clinic and on follow-up appointments and methods of making those appointments. The intent was to learn of the impact of these practices on both the providers and the patients.

Outcome measures   The effects of the educational program on compliance were to be measured in terms of appointment keeping, medication taking, and diet. Blood pressure control as the outcome of the total treatment program was considered the "bottom-line" indicator that patient behaviors had been changed.[16]

The blood pressure measurements and appointment-keeping data as well as other physical and demographic data were derived from medical records. Deciding on a reliable way to measure medication taking required exploration.

Pill counts at the home of the patient were meaningless as a measure for hospital outpatients because patients go to a number of drugstores; patients' pill bottles are refilled before the previous supply is used up; pharmacies may not label consistently; patients may pour pills from one bottle into another; and physicians may change prescriptions, making it difficult to match the right prescription in the medical record with the current prescription the patient is supposed to be following.[17]

Compliance studies have utilized tracers, urine tests, and blood tests to establish disparities between patient reporting on drug regimens and actual behavior.[18] Devoting resources to establishing the degree of imprecision of patient reporting may be useful and acceptable to research studies; however, it may not be considered acceptable in ongoing clinical or community programs, particularly if the encouragement of self-management and acceptance of responsibility are among the stated goals for patient education programs.

In spite of its problems, we decided to use self-reporting as a measure of medication-taking behavior and developed a series of five questions about the behavior.[19] As another facet of the patient baseline survey, we established a locally standardized criterion of blood pressure control.[20]

The provider survey: reinforcing factors   The instrument used in the provider baseline survey was based on a short-term study conducted in the Hopkins Hospital by Inui. After an educational intervention, physicians in an experimental group were found to know more about hypertension, to form higher estimates of the prevalence of noncompliant behavior among patients, and to allocate more patient-visit time to "educational" activities.[21] Because these outcomes were seen as important to producing better patient compliance and control, a modified replication of that study was proposed for this project.

A self-administered questionnaire explored providers' perceptions of some of the enabling and reinforcing factors affecting patient compliance and blood pressure control. It was given to 136 physicians, house staff, and nurses at Hopkins general medical and hypertension clinics. Of these, 46 percent responded. Compared with Inui's survey conducted in the same clinics two years earlier,[22] the staff was found to have relatively accurate knowledge about the diagnosis, management, complications, and preventive aspects of hypertension. Hypertension with poor patient compliance and control was seen as a frequent and significant problem in the clinic, but about one-fourth of the providers estimated that the majority of hypertensive patients in the clinic were under adequate control. Compliance with appointment keeping and prescribed-drug regimens was somewhat overestimated but not as much as in earlier surveys in this hospital and elsewhere. The providers reported spending about 10–15 percent of their visit time on education and counseling functions, and this percentage was higher on follow-up visits. They blamed patient ignorance particularly regarding the asymptomatic nature of the disease and the need for periodic follow-up. Noncompliance in patients was attributed primarily to problems of inconvenience, cost, and travel and secondarily to the fact that patients frequently did not feel ill.

In summary, providers were quite knowledgeable about hypertension as a public health problem and reported devoting effort to educating patients about management. They appreciated the problem of patient noncompliance but attributed it mainly to problems of cost and inconvenience.

The original plan of the project was to follow the diagnostic baseline surveys of patients and providers with continuing education programs directed at staff, to inform them of what patients needed to know and what they needed to do to educate their patients. This plan was dropped. There was little that these surveys revealed that staff did not already suspect; and little change could result from the new information.[23] Our diagnosis was that no major provider education was needed.

Analysis of the system of care: enabling factors Before educational interventions could be initiated, it was necessary to analyze the hospital system for its present effect and potential for change. Just as the providers can have an important effect on the patients, so can the system. The way services are organized and presented, the priorities, the timing of appointments, and the reception of patients all will affect patients' behavior. Providers and patients can have an effect on the system as well. Patients have access to other delivery sites within the hospital and can adopt patterns of use that are not necessarily approved or anticipated by the organization. If physicians and nurses suddenly gave priority to the consistent identification and treatment follow-up of all persons with elevated blood pressures, would the present system be able to accommodate the influx?

This question was studied by means of Emergency Services data. Emergency Services is one access point for new patients and is also used by patients who are already receiving care at other sites. A two-week examination of the patients presenting for care in the emergency room found that 23 percent of them had elevated blood pressures. Based on certain assumptions about the number who might be diagnosed as hypertensive on reexamination, the number already identified and receiving care, and the number who might keep their appointments and continue treatment, estimates were made of new demands for service. The estimates, thought to be realistic but conservative were for a minimum of twenty-six new hypertension patients every week. Fifteen hundred new patients a year would be a 35–40 percent increase over the present clinic population. This number of patients would clearly overload the system and very likely result in less adequate care for the present patients. The system might be able to handle such an influx by decreasing multiple use of facilities, achieving better control of patient flow, and utilizing new mixes of staff, but such steps require time, attention, and additional resources.[24]

The findings from the patient and the provider surveys led to the decision to concentrate the study on the patients in the general medical and hypertension specialty clinics and to continue to discuss potential changes in the care system for future projects.

Baseline survey of the patients: predisposing factors Patients were surveyed by means of interviews. They were questioned about their general knowledge of hypertension as well as about their knowledge of their own regimens. They were also questioned regarding their attitudes and beliefs about the disease; perceived needs for information; perceptions of their family's information and support (reinforcing factors); satisfaction with the services and the providers; problems with side effects; and their problems with transportation, costs, and appointment keeping, and referral (enabling factors). The questions were based on the Health Belief Model and the Health Locus of Control as well as on compliance findings from previously reported studies.[25]

Blood pressure readings and prescribed medical regimens were taken from clinical records.

Patients surveyed in the baseline study were 87 percent black and 69 percent female. Their median age was fifty-five. Median income was reported in the $3,000–$3,400 range; approximately 69 percent were unemployed or retired, and 56 percent were receiving medical assistance benefits. Nearly 60 percent had less than ten years of formal schooling.[26]

Of the 290 patients in the baseline sample whose medical records could be analyzed, elevated blood pressure in 49 percent of the subjects was controlled and in 51 percent was not. These figures matched the widely cited national estimate that blood pressure in 50 percent of hypertensive patients under treament is not adequately controlled.

There were no significant differences in blood pressure control between patients in the general medical clinic and those in the hypertension specialty clinic; between those who kept their last appointment and those who did not; between males and females; between blacks and whites; among groups with differing levels of knowledge about their blood pressure problems or their management; or among groups with varying beliefs in the benefits of treatment.[27]

The only meaningful correlates of blood pressure control at the time of the baseline survey were (1) complexity of drug regimen (the greater the number of drugs prescribed for patients, the less likely they were to meet the criterion of blood pressure control); and an overall compliance score based on patients' verbal reports. The higher the level of self-reported compliance, the lower the clinic-measured blood pressure. The association between complexity of drug regimen and inadequate blood pressure control was the first indication of an educational problem.

The baseline survey found patients' levels of knowledge to be higher than expected relative to a national survey of adults in the general population and relative to the study completed nearly two years earlier in the same clinics. However, the correlations between knowledge and compliance were negligible, even slightly negative.[28]

The percentage of patients responding correctly to most of the specific questions was greater than 80 percent; very few items had less than 50 percent correct-response rates, and none of these would influence compliance significantly. Most patients were well informed, apparently because of the combined effect of the National High Blood Pressure Education Program and other sources of recent publicity about hypertension, patients' awareness of the severity of the disease, and increased medical interest. However, either there had not been enough time for the new beliefs and higher levels of knowledge to influence behavior or there were other barriers to compliance to which health education must be addressed.[29]

We found little correlation between elements of the Health Belief Model and compliance. Neither belief in the *seriousness* of hypertension nor belief in the *benefits* of therapeutic and preventive measures for hypertension and stroke was sufficiently associated with compliance or blood pressure control to justify directing educational programs at changing these beliefs. Interestingly, black patients had much less confidence in the efficacy of treatment (belief in benefits) than whites, but this difference was not reflected in compliance behavior.

Both the survey and less formal comments from patients revealed three influences that shaped decisions on the structure and phasing of educational interventions. First, despite general understanding, patients were confused about their own regimens. Second, patients reported that the support they received from their families was variable. Third, patients showed tendencies to feel dismayed and defeated about not being able to comply or to control their blood pressure.

As further aids to the definition and analysis of the factors affecting compliance behavior, the problems of these patients were discussed with clinic staff, and the patients were observed during the phasing in of the initial interventions. The observations were documented in the open-ended questions and "comment" sections throughout the interview or remembered as observations by the interview staff. Planned debriefing sessions carried out after patient interviews helped to bring these observations into clearer focus and ensure that they were recorded systematically.[30]

When it is not possible to find standard diagnostic instruments appropriate to the problem under study, when no work has been done in the area, or when the situation is in flux, clinical judgment must be exercised and behavioral theory applied to supplement and strengthen the needs-assessment phase. Methodologies to ensure that clinical observations and open-ended inquiries are systematic and objective are illustrated in the literature on ethnomethodology and grounded theory.[31]

Synthesizing clinical observations, theory, and the findings of the survey produced educational diagnostic insights. Several examples of how this worked follow.

Individual regimens: enabling factors   There was a discrepancy between the general level of knowledge these patients had about hypertension and the considerable confusion that was informally noted in relation to their specific regimens. The survey indicated misunderstanding of number of pills, doses per day, hours or timing in relation to meals, and the specific dietary restrictions. Patients could correctly *recognize* facts about their treatment, but they had difficulty *recalling* specific instructions and operationally defining their compliance task. To combat this problem, patients' personal regimens were reviewed with them immediately after physicians issued or renewed prescriptions. Patients received personalized attention rather than a standardized informational package such as would normally accompany an educational program. Clinical observations, combined with the recognition from theory that behavioral change requires a high degree of specificity, personal relevance, and a concrete behavioral focus, led to setting up procedures for an exit interview with each patient that would address the problem.

Family support: reinforcing factors   Patients were asked in the baseline survey whether they expected or generally received any help from family members in complying with their medical regimens. There were major differences in positive responses, for example, between males (83 percent) and females (65 percent); and between patients on sodium-restriction regimens (64 percent) and those on weight-reduction regimens (82 percent). From a review of the literature on the roles family members play in compliance of patients, we were convinced that this was a neglected dimension of health education with great potential.[32]

In the course of interviews, patients' formal responses to our questions indicated that they would like members of their families to know more about hypertension and would welcome educational materials that they could take home. They did not specifically claim, however, that family members were unsupportive or not helpful to them in controlling their blood pressure. Again, rather than addressing the problem by merely transferring general information about hypertension to family members, we leaned on the behavioral interpretation of the clinical observation to develop an intervention that would result in families' receiving specific suggestions on how they could help their own hypertensive family member. An educational pamphlet was prepared to be reviewed with family members during home visits. Space in the pamphlet was provided for writing down specific ways in which family members could support the diet or medication regimen of the specific hypertensive patient. Again, the specificity and relevance of the information and the expected behavior made this intervention more appropriate than one we might have designed on the basis of the survey data alone.[33]

Self-confidence in regimen: predisposing factor   Another major observation that influenced our interpretation of the statistical data and our development of the interventions was the discrepancy between the positive attitudes that patients expressed about the value of their treatment and their willingness to follow their medical regimens and their feelings of defeat and despair. Either their attitudinal responses were merely passive or they were experiencing considerable dissonance between what they wanted to do and what they found themselves able to do. The discrepancy was interpreted according to behavioral theory as a problem of locus of control.[34] An intervention was designed with the aim of building patients' self-confidence in their ability to manage their regimens. Small-group discussions with other patients were thought to be the most effective vehicle for reinforcing expressions of success and control and analyzing shared problems in attaining blood pressure control.

The baseline study included questions about such enabling factors as transportation, costs, barriers to care, and satisfaction with the system of care. Few of the variations reported in the perceptions of availability and accessibility to the system correlated with behavior or blood pressure control.

The original plan to follow the baseline surveys with continuing education programs for staff was modified greatly because of the educational diagnosis. It became clear that had we proceeded on the basis of theory and reported experience alone we would have wasted our resources and produced, in the bargain, ineffective educational programs. The diagnostic survey enabled us to target the educational programs to the appropriate enabling, reinforcing and predisposing factors. Our approach was one of holding to a plan in which the logic, design, and desired outcomes were structured, but the content and method of the specific educational interventions were left open, subject to testing and review.

The revised plan was to direct the intervention experiments to the three areas of problems identified. Then on the basis of the results from these trials, a clinical package that could be used and adapted by the regular personnel in the clinic would be constructed.

It was not the purpose of the project to produce behavior change under circumstances that could not be readily replicated. Thus, a characteristic of the interventions was that they could be carried out by regular clinic personnel in the ongoing daily procedure. For this project, however, personnel were added. Until the efficacy of the interventions was proven, disruption of the busy clinics could not be justified.

To summarize, the hypotheses generated through the needs-assessment stage posited the need for enabling and clarifying individual regimens, generating social support, and building patients' self-confidence. The interventions were to be initiated in an order beginning with the least complicated and least expensive and ending with the most complicated.

The Design of the Program and the Interventions Used

The 400 patients who participated in the experimental program, including 350 who received various combinations of educational interventions and 50 in a control group, were a different sample selected from the same pool of patients as those in the baseline survey. Patients in both samples had similar demographic, social, and disease characteristics. They were 91 percent black and 70 percent female. They had a median age of fifty-four, a median income of $3,250 and a median of seven years of formal schooling. The average time they had been treated for hypertension was six years; the range was from six months to eighteen years. Using an age-adjusted criterion for blood pressure control, 40 percent were found to have their blood pressure under control.

The three educational interventions provided are described briefly below. More detailed explanations can be found in papers published and presented on this project.[35]

Phase 1: Exit interview in the clinic – reteaching-reinforcement Individualized reteaching and reinforcement sessions following patient-practitioner encounters in general medical and hypertension clinics were provided to 200 patients during March–May 1975. The purpose of the 20-minute sessions was to go over the specific instructions given by providers relative to medication schedules, diet, and return visits. Trained graduate health education students using clock and calendar aids adapted patients' medication regimens to their own daily schedules. They referred patients to other hospital resources and outside agencies for nonclinical problems such as finances, housing, and employment.

Phase 2: Household reinforcement The second intervention combined the characteristics of a home visit with behavior reinforcement in an effort to influence members of patients' households. Patients from the control and experimental groups who participated in the phase-1 intervention were interviewed June–September 1975 concerning their knowledge and attitudes about hypertension, treatment regimens, and compliance behavior. In addition, each was asked to identify the person in his or her household who had the most potential for providing behavioral reinforcement for the patient. Each of the people selected was sought out for a separate interview and given specific information on hypertension and on what the patient was to do. Suggestions on how to help a patient comply were also given.

Phase 3: Small-group discussions Small-group discussions, the third intervention, took place March–June 1976. Their purpose was to provide support to patients lacking self-confidence through discussions centering on hypertension management and compliance. Random sets of sixteen patients were recruited to group discussions and asked to return for a total of three sessions, each lasting an hour and a half. The content of the groups was specified and analyzed so that the intervention could be replicated by discussion leaders from several disciplines and at other times. Group sessions included a broad range of short-term, mostly action-oriented, procedures (role playing, behavior rehearsal, problem clarification, cognitive restructuring). Organization of the group sessions was such as would move patients toward more self-direction in dealing with their medical situations. The theoretical process that guided measurement of intermediate outcomes for this intervention was reinforcement of locus of control.[36] Patients were to strengthen their perceptions of themselves as able to cope with and control their own problems related to blood pressure.

After the interventions were completed, the patients were interviewed in their homes once more to collect information on their knowledge, attitudes, and behavior. Their records were reviewed to collect medical information, blood pressure recordings, and information on appointment keeping and weight.

RESULTS OF THE PROGRAM

The program produced a favorable effect on blood pressure control. The group of patients assigned to all three of the interventions achieved 66 percent control in contrast to the 38 percent control they had previously; the rate of control for the control group, who received none of the interventions, remained unchanged at 42 percent. The percentage of change is shown in table B.3.

There were also improvements in the proportion of patients losing weight (56 percent in the experimental group versus 35 percent in the control group) and in appointment keeping (76 percent in the experiment group versus 63 percent in the control group). The control group and the experimental group showed little difference in adherence to salt-restricted diets. In terms of appointment keeping, two intervention combinations produced statistically significant improvements over the control group. These were: the home visit–family support intervention and the exit interview; and the exit interview and small-group discussions.

Analysis showed that the decreases found in the proportion of patients with moderate or severe hypertension were maintained over a period of time ranging up to eighteen months. This pattern of consistently improved compliance and blood pressure control in the clinic population who received the interventions cannot be accounted for on the basis of a single marked behav-

TABLE B.3
Percentage of patients with blood pressures under control, by study status

Intervention status	Before program (%)	After program (%)	Change (%)	Number
Control ($C_1C_2C_3$)	41	42	+ 1	40
Exit interview only	40	41	+ 1	46
Family support only	37	48	+11	42
Small group only	34	52	+18	44
Exit interview and small group	40	53	+13	47
Family support and small group	41	54	+13	43
Exit interview and family support	45	55	+10	44
Exit interview, family support, and small group	38	66	+28	44
All experimental groups combined	40	52	+12	310

SOURCE: Adapted from D. M. Levine et al., "Health Education for Hypertensive Patients," *Journal of American Medical Association* 241 (April 20, 1979): 1700–1703.

ior change. The interventions appear to have had a multiple accumulative low-level effect that could not be detected by analysis of any one output.[37]

It is not clear why the combination of interventions had such an effect. Either the total package acted synergistically or the effect was due to factors influencing blood pressure control that were not investigated in the study. Certainly replication of the study with larger samples would be helpful in clarifying cause-effect relationships.

Every health program design is a compromise between the best, most-individualized approach and what the organization can afford. In addition to demonstrating a systematic method of planning and designing educational activities, we have throughout this case study attempted to show how that compromise is reached. It is a result of gathering data, sorting them out, reaching tentative conclusions, and then revising on the basis of additional data collected during the pilot phases of implementation. Resulting health education strategies reflect a perspective in which certain general educational approaches are directed toward commonalities in a particular group. The general educational approach is then individualized as much as possible within the limits of available resources. Inevitably this results in a compromise between efficiency and effectiveness, but such a compromise as we have been discussing here is both respectable and rational.

APPENDIX C
Student Applications of the PRECEDE Framework

IN THE DEPARTMENTS of health education at the Johns Hopkins School of Hygiene and Public Health and the College of Health at the University of Utah, we have used PRECEDE both as a general planning framework for curriculum development and as a content base for specific courses in health education program planning and evaluation. In these courses, we typically ask students to use the PRECEDE framework to prepare mock applications for grants to aid them in developing, implementing, and evaluating experimental health education programs. Depending on the students' specialties and interests, they are asked to form interdisciplinary "teams" of three. A variety of health-care providers, administrators, physicians, nurses, social workers, and health education specialists may be represented.

Prepared in 1978 by Zoe Clayson, Peggy McManus, Ariel Miller, and Mariquita Mullan, Johns Hopkins University; material edited for this book and notes omitted.

211

Proposals follow the basic phases of PRECEDE. A program or project is justified in terms of the social and epidemiologic diagnoses. The program objectives are then spelled out, followed by a rather detailed discussion of specific behaviors (behavioral diagnosis) and the factors that are likely to affect those behaviors (educational diagnosis). A description of the educational program is usually presented next, along with an administrative diagnosis identifying potential barriers to and facilitators of program success. The proposals conclude with a concrete research design, recommendations for evaluation procedures, and a hypothetical budget.

We are impressed by the facility with which our students apply the planning model and the high caliber of their work. To illustrate the potential application of PRECEDE in an academic setting, we want to share excerpts from four student projects submitted in 1978. A brief description of each proposal is followed by application of selected phases of the PRECEDE framework to the proposed project.

PROPOSAL 1—INDUSTRIAL WORKERS' HEALTH AND POLITICAL EDUCATION PROGRAM PROPOSAL FOR UNITED STEELWORKERS UNION

Proposal 1 details a creative educational and political approach to occupational health problems and hazards for steelworkers. Political and social action form the bases for its orientation; the educational intervention is directed primarily to management behaviors and the question of how workers can best affect management's action. Two excerpts are presented here. In the first excerpt, the students have creatively modified the PRECEDE framework to fit their specific objectives. The second excerpt presents the educational diagnosis of the workers.

Rationale for the Program

The following proposal outlines an educational intervention that has as its ultimate objective reducing the incidence of occupational illnesses and accidents. Occupational diseases come about when workers are exposed to toxic substances in the work place; workers have accidents when they are exposed to dangerous situations.

The degree to which workers are exposed to hazards of both kinds is in essence a function of behavior, particularly the behavior of management vis-à-vis the following elements of production:

1. *Choice of substances to be used in production*—use of substances with acute or long-term toxic effects creates the possibility of hazardous exposure.
2. *Design of machinery*—inadequate design of machinery is a major factor affecting the probability of hazardous emissions or accidents.
3. *Implementation of effective controls of hazards*—a hierarchy of controls can be applied to reduce or eliminate an occupational hazard. Some are more effective than others, and management's choice of a control method has a profound effect on the degree to which workers are exposed to hazards.
4. *Work practices*—work practices such as the assignment of workers to hazardous areas and the length of the shifts govern: (*a*) the number of people exposed to a hazard and (*b*) the duration of the exposure. Hence, they affect the incidence of disease and accidents.
5. *Maintenance and upkeep* of machinery and safety devices—maintenance and upkeep are important determinants of the degree to which hazards are controlled over time.

Accordingly, management should be a prime target of efforts to bring about effective control of industrial hazards. To identify the type of intervention most likely to succeed in changing management's policies on the prevention of disease and accidents, we have carried out an educational diagnosis of the predisposing, enabling, and reinforcing factors in management's behavior. The following key factors affecting management behavior seem to be amenable to change through educational interventions:

1. management's awareness of the existence of occupational hazards
2. management's perception of the cost of controlling them (a powerful incentive related to the desire to minimize costs of production and maximize profits)

Potential agents for changing these perceptions are:

1. regulatory agencies, through setting of standards, inspection, enforcement, and adjudication
2. workers, through collective action
3. insurance companies, through adjustments in health insurance premiums
4. health educators, through persuasive communications and technical assistance
5. public opinion and press coverage, through expressions of good will or disapproval

Collective action by workers seems to have the greatest potential for inducing management to bring about more effective controls. Regulatory

FIGURE C.1A
Analysis and program design

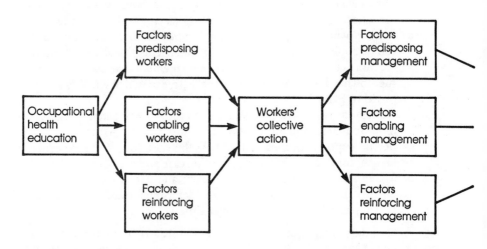

agencies such as OSHA (Occupational Safety and Health Administration) have undoubtedly contributed to improvements in working conditions, but their effectiveness is greatly hampered by the limited penalties permitted under law, the cumbersomeness of standards setting and enforcement procedures, and the shortage of qualified staff. Only a handful of standards has been set in the eight years since the passage of the OSHA Act, even though over 5,000 substances used in industry are known to be hazardous. The staff of OSHA (like the staff of other regulatory agencies) is small and simply unable to inspect the thousands of separate work areas subject to the OSHA Act.

Press coverage and public outcry are intermittent phenomena, rarely backed by meaningful economic sanctions such as consumer boycotts. Insurance companies and state workmen's compensation premiums do give management some incentive to control hazards; however, premiums do not reflect the full cost of disease. Further, most occupational diseases are not compensable under state workmen's compensation laws, because they have multiple etiologies, and because the risk attributable to occupational exposure is often neither well documented nor generally accepted. Health educators who try to persuade management directly to clean up the work place are even less likely to be effective, because they lack the power to impose economic and legal sanctions.

Workers, on the other hand, bear the burden of occupational accidents and disease, and thus have a personal stake in prevention. Since labor is essen-

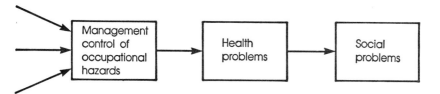

tial to production, collective action by workers can be an effective economic sanction, requiring management to revise its estimates of the cost of occupational disease and accidents. As a strategy, collective action has great potential for increasing management's desire to control occupational hazards.

The intermediate goal of our educational intervention is thus to motivate and enable workers to take effective collective action to improve working conditions. Our analysis and program design proceed according to figure C.1A.

The direct target of our educational efforts is the group of workers employed in a given plant. In designing our intervention we have been advised and encouraged by the members of Local 2609 of the United Steelworkers of America, who work at the Sparrows Point plant of Bethlehem Steel, and have developed a program to meet the needs of this group. The discussion that follows is based on the comments and work situation of these union members.

Description of the Recommended Innovation

In preliminary discussions, we were able to identify several obstacles to collective action directed toward occupational-health issues, including the following:

1. lack of access to company records, the only existing source of data documenting hazards in the plant
2. a sense of powerlessness arising from the perceived ability of management to retaliate against collective action by laying off or firing workers
3. the perceived weakness of current legal and economic means of bringing about improvements in working conditions

To address these obstacles, our intervention is intended to

1. motivate and enable workers to collect and maintain their own records of work hazards
2. acquaint workers with legal and economic remedies available to them
3. inform workers of the successes of other unions in bargaining for improvements in working conditions
4. reinforce workers in designing and carrying out collective-action strategies

A work hazard surveillance system will be developed for the collection of epidemiologic and environmental data. Documentation of excess risk of accidents or diseases related to occupational exposure must include records of the names and characteristics of the population at risk. In many industries, as in steelmaking, many processes go on in a single plant, and workers performing different jobs are subject to different exposures. Rosters of the population at risk must be maintained for each distinct work area in the plant. Essential data are:

1. Sex, race, date of birth, and ethnic background of every worker— those demographic variables affect health status and are needed for adjustment purposes in isolating the effect of occupation on health.
2. Dates of entering and leaving employment in particular work areas —length of employment by work area is used as a proxy for the duration of exposure. Many diseases, including most cancers, exhibit a dose-response relationship. As a result, to get accurate measures of risk it is essential to examine incidence rates by exposure category. Failure to distinguish short-term from long-term exposure can lead to a spurious conclusion of no excess risk.

To document the nature of hazardous exposures and to monitor the effectiveness of controls implemented to reduce them, workers will need to gather data on certain facets of the environment.

1. Substances used—a historical record should be kept of all substances used in production, by trade name and chemical composition.

2. Emissions or hazardous work processes—descriptions of these hazards should be recorded as they arise and kept as a historical record.
3. Controls implemented—types of controls should be described and their date of implementation recorded. Continuous surveillance of their effectiveness should be carried out, and findings recorded in a log.

This information is essential to relating exposures or hazardous conditions to accidents or excess disease in the population at risk. Without it, one can only hypothesize about the causes of excess illness or accidents, and the design of effective controls is accordingly hampered. Thus, the goals of the educational program are:

1. to train workers to carry out epidemiologic and environmental surveillance in every work area, to keep continuous records, and to seek professional advice when necessary in evaluating the data
2. to encourage and equip workers to use the information they collect as a basis for collective action

For educational purposes workers are divided into two groups. One group will consist of monitors who will be elected by work area and trained to carry out surveillance and record keeping. The other will consist of workers at large, who will make decisions to take collective action on given issues.

The goals and objectives of the program are outlined on figure C.1B. Here, we discuss social and health problems resulting from occupational hazards and the educational diagnosis of workers.

Social Problems

Because of inadequate reporting and compensation of occupationally related disease, the exact extent and magnitude of social problems caused directly or indirectly by occupational hazards and disease is unknown. Estimates have been made of a number of costs, however. These estimates are undoubtedly low and are offered as a conservative assessment of the size of the problem.

Overall costs

1. The National Safety Council, in 1971, estimated that about $9.3 billion—nearly 1 percent of the gross national product—was lost in terms of wages, medical expenses, insurance claims, production delays, lost time of co-workers, and equipment damage due to occupational illness and accidents. Premature death and retirement, reduced efficiency, and family and community problems are not included in this estimate.

FIGURE C.1B

Goals and objectives in reducing the incidence of occupational diseases and accidents at Bethlehem Steel's Sparrows Point plant

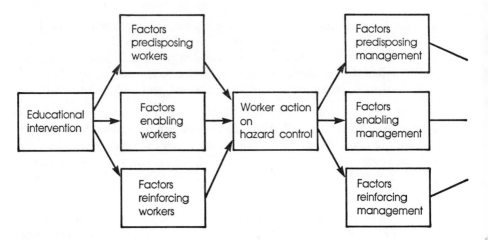

Worker Educational Objectives

Within one year of the training program, two monitors per work shift per work area will

1. demonstrate basic skills in industrial hygiene monitoring
2. demonstrate knowledge of patho-physiology related to occupational exposures
3. demonstrate knowledge of legal remedies available
4. carry out the monitoring and record keeping described as part of behavioral objectives
5. be responsible for training new monitors

Within two years, 50 percent of the workers in the plant will

6. demonstrate knowledge of occupational hazards.
7. same as 2 and 3

Worker Behavioral Objectives

1. To implement monitoring and surveillance in each work area within one year
2. To establish a hazards record and personnel-assignment log in each work area within one year and to maintain it over time
3. To formulate demands for management to improve hazardous conditions
4. To take collective action to compel management to improve conditions in the work place.

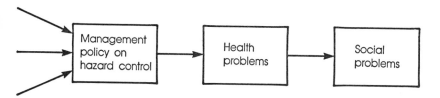

Management Behavioral Objectives	Health Goals	Social Goals
1. To recognize and acknowledge the existence of each hazard 2. To institute controls that will reliably eliminate or minimize risk 3. To maintain the controls in good working order	For each occupational disease discovered by surveillance: To reduce incidence by x percent within y years after the source of the causative exposure is discovered and controlled (where x = the excess risk attributable to the exposure and y = the latency of the disease)	1. To reduce incidence of: Absenteeism Lost wages Medical expenses Workmen's compensation claims Production loss and delays Early retirement 2. To prevent the "intangible" effects of occupational disease: Anguish and pain Loss of workers' and families' financial independence Mistrust between workers and management

2. An estimated 25 million workdays were lost through absenteeism during 1972. This figure is equivalent to a loss of 100,000 person-years of work.
3. In 1970, workmen's compensation cost employers $4.9 billion, 1.13 percent of covered payrolls.

Population exposed to potential hazards

1. The Surgeon General reported to Congress in 1968 that an estimated 65 percent of industrial workers were "exposed to toxic materials or harmful physical agent. Of these, only 25½ were adequately safeguarded."
2. Dr. Joseph Wagoner of the National Institute of Occupational Safety and Health reported that industrial workers suffer a disproportionately higher occupational disease rate than the general employed population.

Human suffering—The University of Michigan conducted, in 1973, a survey on behalf of the Department of Labor. Of workers interviewed, 41 percent reported health and safety hazards on the job, and 42 percent reported having lost two or more weeks a year of work for this reason. Two-thirds of this group reported difficulty in meeting medical and living expenses while out of work due to occupational disease.

These figures relate to only a few of the social problems caused by occupational hazards. Others include air and water pollution, worker alienation, and social disintegration. All must be considered in the planning, implementation, and evaluation of occupational health education programs.

Health Problems

Occupational disease in the United States is reaching epidemic proportions. The Public Health Service estimates that 390,000 new cases of occupational disease occur annually. Nicholas Ashford states that as many as 100,000 deaths each year are occupationally related. Actuarial data compiled by insurance companies indicates that the risk of death in certain occupational groups is greater than twice that of a matched cohort from the general population. For example, asbestos workers have a 2.6-fold greater risk of lung cancer than the general population. Workers exposed to vinyl chloride have twice the risk of cancer; benzene workers, two to three times the risk of leukemia; and nickel workers, 100 times the general population risk of cancer of the nasal passage, sinuses, and lung. Coke workers have been found to have significant excess mortality from cancer of several sites compared to steelworkers who were never employed in coke plants.

Educational Diagnosis of Workers – Initial Impressions

We have sat in on informal discussions among steelworkers on the merits and drawbacks of a worker-controlled surveillance system and collective action to improve safety in the work place. Their comments are a major source for the list of predisposing, reinforcing, and enabling factors presented in table C.1A. The factors are ranked in table C.1B.

David Wilson, president of Local 2609 of the United Steelworkers; a young member of a local at Armco Steel; and an older worker from the Sparrows Point plant took part in these discussions. All three believe that occupational disease is a real hazard in steelmaking in Baltimore. They mentioned clusters of cancer, pulmonary disease, and heart disease associated with clearly dangerous conditions in specific work places. The worker-controlled surveillance system was seen as a potentially valuable way to document hazards. But there were thought to be many impediments to its effective implementation and use as a tool for change, including attitudes of individual susceptible workers. Many of the workers at Sparrows Point have been employed there for at least twenty years. They do not believe that chronic diseases such as cancer are preventable after so many years of exposure. Further, younger workers are not greatly impressed by the risk of disease many years in the future, and they are little motivated to monitor work environments. In addition, many workers do not want to know that they are at risk of cancer (which is considered a death sentence) or other chronic diseases. This desire, which is particularly strong in workers with several years' exposure who plan to spend the rest of their working lives in the steel plant, is seen as a major obstacle to the implementation of a worker-controlled surveillance system.

Generally speaking, it is very hard for local union members to do anything to compel management to institute effective control of hazards. However, when a hazard is really obvious, workers are apt to acknowledge it and demand that it be controlled. Several instances of such action were described.

One of the chief drawbacks to the use of collective action to seek improvements in working conditions is seen to be the inadequacy of channels available to workers. This inadequacy is reflected in a number of areas. The Maryland Occupational Health and Safety Administration is considered particularly ineffectual in bringing about improvements in conditions that affect health. Further, the parent union, United Steelworkers of America, has not taken a strong position on occupational health and discourages activism by the locals on this issue. The Safety and Health Committee of the parent union described its own actions as "firefighting." Rather than working for the prevention of hazards, the union reacts to isolated cases as they develop, seeking compensation for the worker. A member of the Safety and Health Committee admitted to David Wilson that it had not considered asking the company for work histories or medical records of union members and that it did not feel it had the capability to collect and maintain such records on its own.

Striking is, of course, a possibility, but at Sparrows Point a remote one. The parent union has negotiated a contract with the steel industry that in-

---

TABLE C.1A

Workers: Predisposing, enabling, and reinforcing factors

Predisposing factors

Empowerment-related beliefs
1. Isolated individualism: "What I do doesn't matter."
2. "The union is ineffective and wouldn't support me."
3. "Management is invulnerable."
4. "Regulatory agencies are powerless and ineffective."
5. "Politicians [substitute *organized crime,* etc.] control everything."
6. Self-evaluation: "I'm no good because I'm only a factory worker and if I were any good I would be rich."
7. Worker satisfaction/alienation: "Everyone hates his job, but there is no other choice. That's just the price we pay for industrialization" [or technology, progress, and civilization, etc.].

Knowledge and attitudes
1. There is a high level of awareness of occupational-disease risk (confirmed by pretest interviews). Fear of cancer (as a death sentence) and feeling that there is no alternative to accepting such working conditions could cause a rejection of information.
2. Knowledge received previously through traditional education, church, media, and peers relative to political economy, history, and social analyses may be contradictory; or there may be none.
3. Health/legal information is reserved for specialists. Workers feel that they do not have sufficient background to understand.

Collective consciousness
1. Cultural hegemony regarding issues of individualism, victim blaming, competiveness, hierarchical division of labor, and communism is pervasive.
2. Groups need to feel superior to each other.
3. Differences are feared.
4. Sexual/racial stereotyping prevails.
5. Capitalist economy fosters sexism and racism as tools to divide the working class.

Enabling factors

Economic security—As a threat of economic recession increases, workers become more afraid of losing their jobs and hence more afraid to confront management. Objectively, conditions in industry make it easy to replace workers by increasing compartmentalized, unskilled detail work in production

cludes a no-strike provision in effect until 1983. Locals can strike on local issues only if a number of conditions are met, one of which is a majority vote among members of the plant that the issue is strikeable. Sparrows Point workers belong to two locals, one of which (2610) is reluctant to act on occu-

---

processes. Historically, worker demands for increased wages and improved working conditions motivated technological innovations by industry to displace greater numbers of workers. Management certainly tries to get rid of troublemakers first. Without strong union support an individual might be fined, demoted, laid off, or fired.

Convenience of program—Attendance at activities at the union hall may be inconvenient because of the times scheduled for activities and the location of the union hall.

Collective action by workers—Existing contracts may have issue-limiting clauses, no-strike clauses, and inadequate grievance procedure or workers' right-to-know mechanisms.

Educational format
1. There may not be enough materials or materials of the right kind.
2. Presentations and formulations may not conceptualize reality (real conditions and life experiences of the workers).

Reinforcing factors

Commitment by union
1. Union leaders look after their own interests; for example, union leadership has traditionally tried to proceduralize all worker demands.
2. Union leaders may see this program as necessary only if it ensures that they will not be sued by sick employees.
3. Local may get pressure from international leadership or from the AFL/CIO lobby to "lay off" the issue.

Commitment by family
1. Families may have economic fears, that they will lose their homes and that they won't be able to survive.
2. There may be social pressures around the belief that political analysis is un-American and around the fear of losing friends and peer status and a general fear of the unknown.

Sensitivity and ability of health educator
1. Previous interaction with workers may be lacking.
2. The educator may not be adequately prepared.
3. The educator may be biased; for example, he or she may believe that all Americans are either middle or upper class or that health does not relate to politics.
4. The self-image of the educator may not be facilitating, as would be the case if a strong sense of credibility and legitimacy were missing.

pational health issues for fear that the company will lay off certain exposed workers in retaliation. David Wilson's observation is that the company lays off workers primarily for economic reasons, not as punishment for specific actions by the union, but that it encourages the local to believe that layoffs are in retaliation for activism.

Grievance procedures, a usual means of seeking redress, can only be used to protest company violations of contract provisions. Furthermore, they are extremely slow. Arbitration can take as long as a year and a half.

Ironically, Local 2609 is also hampered in its ability to mobilize workers by its own success in representing them on this and other issues. Confidence in the local leadership translates into low attendance at meetings. When political controversy is high in the local or immediate problems are not being effectively handled, attendance figures are much higher and it is easier to collect an audience for educational purposes. At present, local members may have a somewhat misled sense of progress because the local leadership has a productive relationship with elected officials, good and frequent press coverage, and easy access to professional advice from the Johns Hopkins medical institutions. It may be difficult to get the attention of and motivate a sufficient number of workers to carry out a training program and have workers set up a monitoring system in each work area.

TABLE C.1B
Ranking of predisposing, enabling, and reinforcing factors for workers

Importance

	High	Low
High	1. Belief about disease 2. Collective consciousness 3. Empowerment-related beliefs 4. Educational format 5. Family commitment	1. Union commitment 2. Convenience of program 3. Ability of educator
Changeability Low	1. Economic security	This quadrant does not apply.

NOTE: It is extremely difficult to "rank" these factors without additional confirmation of our hypotheses. In addition, the goals considered are all interrelated and equally important. To permanently rank these factors without dialogue with workers is to negate the collective process itself. Workers would be dealt with as objects (those who are known *and* acted on) rather than as subjects (those who know *and* act.)

The matrix attempts, then, with severe reservations, to make use of the changeability and importance method of ranking.

PROPOSAL 2 – PHYSICIAN EDUCATION COMPONENT OF A
CHILD-ABUSE PREVENTION PROGRAM

In this proposal, the problem of child abuse is approached from the point of view that the most effective educational intervention must begin with the education of health-care providers. In the excerpt given here, Cohen and her colleagues present behavioral and educational diagnoses of health-care providers as these in turn influence parental behavior.

Rationale for the Program

Hometown has a number of programs dealing with factors that predispose parents to abusive behavior, among them drug abuse and alcoholism programs and mental health clinics. Treatment programs directed toward reinforcing behavioral change among abusive parents are also available. These programs, designed to meet the dependency needs of the parents and to introduce the parents to new behaviors and attitudes regarding child rearing, also address enabling factors such as lack of parenting skills and social isolation and reinforcing factors involving the family and significant others.

The intention of this program is to focus on behaviors exhibited by health-care workers that may serve to reinforce changes in the behavior of abusive parents. Sometimes, for example, the negative attitudes of physicians toward abusers are exhibited in terms of condemnatory accusations. This approach almost ensures that families will not return children to hospitals or private offices for follow-up visits. Impersonal care and excluding the parents from discussions of the disposition of their children's cases may also cause parents to discontinue treatment. Health workers may fail to familiarize parents with community resources and alternative child-rearing practices. Failure to provide anticipatory guidance and to predict children and parents at risk has also been reported. Although there is no isolated predictor of abuse, a series of factors including youth of the parents, emotional disturbance of the parents, expressed concern over suitability for parenthood, and frequent emergency visits can indicate potential for abuse.

When ranked on scales of importance and potential for change, three behaviors of health-care workers, specifically physicians, were thought to be extremely important and, within the scope of an intervention program, highly changeable. These behaviors—discharging abused children to homes inappropriately or without adequate follow-up, failure to report suspected cases of abuse to appropriate agencies, and failure to refer children who are

Prepared in 1978 by Colleen Roach, Laurie Liskin, and Janet Cohen, Johns Hopkins University; material edited for this book and notes omitted.

suspected victims of abuse to appropriate resources—are the target of the behavioral objectives of this program.

Behaviors of physicians are ranked in table C.2A according to their importance and changeability within the context of the community of Hometown.

TABLE C.2A

Behaviors of physicians, reinforcing abusive behavior in parents, ranked according to changeability and importance

Importance	Potential for change	Behavior
High	High	Failure to refer children who are suspected victims of abuse to appropriate resources
High	High	Failure to report suspected cases of child abuse to appropriate agencies
High	High	Discharging the child to home inappropriately or without adequate follow-up
High	Medium	Not including parent in discussion of disposition of the child
Medium	Medium	Providing impersonal care
Medium	Medium	Failure to provide anticipatory guidance
Medium	Medium	Failure to familiarize parents with community resources and alternative child-rearing practices
Medium	Low	Failure to predict children and parents at risk

Predisposing, Enabling, and Reinforcing Factors: Physicians

Because of funding limitations, it is necessary to rank the predisposing, enabling, and reinforcing factors having to do with the behavior of physicians. Doing so makes it possible to direct scarce resources to meeting objectives that are both important and likely to be met successfuly. Rankings,

presented in table C.2B, are based on a review of the literature and on characteristics peculiar to Hometown. For example, although a complex and inefficient referral system would be an important consideration in any child-abuse
program, it is assumed that Hometown's system is adequate and efficient.
Thus, it merits low priority for this particular program.

TABLE C.2B
Ranking of predisposing, enabling, and reinforcing factors: Physicians

Importance	Potential for change	Predisposing factors
High	High	Ignorance of referral and support resources in the community
High	High	Ignorance of signs and symptoms of child abuse
High	High	Ignorance of the dimensions of the child-abuse problem
High	High	Ignorance of child-abuse statutes and legal obligations of the physician
High	High	Belief that nothing can be done to ameliorate the problem
High	High	Belief that relevant referral and support services are inadequate
Medium	Low	Beliefs of physician relevant to child-rearing practices
		Belief that reporting suspected cases of child abuse will lead to
High	High	1. liability
High	High	2. bureaucratic entanglements
High	Low	3. damaged professional reputation
High	Low	4. loss of practice and fees
High	High	Belief that reporting suspected cases of child abuse will further endanger the child
High	Low	Hostile attitude toward abusive parents
High	Medium	Fear of talking with and dealing with angry parents
High	Low	Type of medical specialty to which the physician belongs

TABLE C.2B continued

Importance	Potential for change	Enabling factors
Low	Not applicable in hometown	Complex and/or inefficient referral system and support system
High	Low	Length of time the physician must spend in legal/judicial proceedings
Low	Not applicable in hometown	Relevant community resources not available
High	High	Lack of previous first-hand experience with child-abuse cases and/or inadequate medical education
High	High	Lack of communication skills for dealing with suspected or actual abusers
High	High	Ambiguous diagnostic guidelines
Low	Not applicable in hometown	Lack of institutional support: insufficient time to do thorough evaluation of suspected cases; no funds provided for laboratory screening for suspected cases

Importance	Potential for change	Reinforcing factors
Low	Not applicable in hometown	Complex and/or inefficient referral and support system
High	Low	Community/professional peer pressure: physician in a small community who reports a suspected case of child abuse may be ostracized; peers may try to persuade him or her that it is unwise to "get involved"
High	Medium	Lack of feedback from referral system regarding cases referred
Low	Not applicable in hometown	Consultant services for child-abuse cases not available

We can summarize the factors ranked high both in importance and in changeability. These factors will serve as the basis for the cognitive and attitudinal objectives of the program.

1. physician's knowledge of the referral and resource system, the signs and symptoms of child abuse, the dimensions of the problem, and the child-abuse statutes
2. physician's beliefs that nothing can be done and that services are inadequate
3. physician's concerns about liability and bureaucratic involvements
4. physician's perception of conflicting roles as healer and reporter
5. physician's experience and education
6. physician's communication skills
7. clarity of diagnostic guidelines

Objectives

By gearing objectives toward physicians' knowledge, attitudes, perceptions, and skills, it is anticipated that their diagnostic, reporting, and referring behaviors will improve and that these improvements will, in turn, contribute to success in meeting the overall program objectives of reducing the incidence and prevalence of child abuse and providing better management of diagnosed cases. However, since the team's responsibility is limited, it has as its behavioral objectives the following:

1. The number of cases of suspected child abuse reported by physicians to the Children's Protective Services will increase over last year's figures according to the following schedule:
   a) by 50 percent one year after the program.
   b) by 65 percent two years after the program.
2. The number of cases of suspected child abuse reported by physicians to the pediatric social worker will increase over last year's figures according to the following schedule:
   a) by 20 percent six months after the program.
   b) by 60 percent one year after the program.
3. The number of children under the age of five years admitted to the hospital for any traumatic injury will increase over last year's admission rates according to the following schedule:
   a) by 15 percent six months after the program.
   b) by 35 percent one year after the program.
4. There will be an increase in the number of long bone and skull X rays taken on children under the age of five years according to the following schedule:
   a) by 20 percent six months after the program.
   b) by 50 percent one year after the program.
5. There will be an increase in the number of screening tests (defined)

These behavioral objectives can not be met without focusing on the predisposing and enabling factors that inform them. Intermediate cognitive and attitudinal objectives were thus developed. Achievement of objectives in the cognitive domain and affective domain will be measured by means of a continuing-education pretest and post test approved by the AMA. The post test will be administered three months after the conclusion of the program. The standard of acceptability will be the following: 85 percent of the participating physicians will score 50 percent higher on the post test than they scored on the pretest. Objectives measured by the AMA test are:

1. The physician will be able to demonstrate the technique for communicating to parents that he or she suspects that their child has been abused by selecting from among several statements the one that is most appropriate and therapeutic.
2. The physician will identify the five most common presenting injuries in child abuse.
3. The physician will identify six elements (unexplained injury, discrepant history, alleged self-injury in a small baby, blame on third party, delay in seeking medical care, repeated suspicious injuries) in injury histories that should lead to suspicion of abuse.
4. The physician's fear of and hostility toward abusive parents will diminish when measured on an attitudinal scale.
5. The physician's attitude toward the efficacy of available resources for treatment of child abusers and placement of abused children will improve when measured on an attitudinal scale.
6. The physician's fear of liability, damage to reputation and practice, and bureaucratic entanglements resulting from reporting suspected cases of child abuse will decrease when measured on an attitudinal scale.
7. The physician's concern that reporting a suspected case of child abuse will further endanger the child will be reduced when measured on an attitudinal scale.
8. The physician will exhibit an increased awareness of the dimensions of the child-abuse problem on a national level by:
   a) identifying reported incidence figures.
   b) stating the estimated extent of underreporting.
   c) identifying the child-abuse mortality rates.
   d) identifying the percentage of abused children who sustain permanent disabilities as a result of abuse.

Achievement of objectives in a second set of cognitive outcomes not included in the AMA test will be measured on a questionnaire designed by the team, administered before the beginning of the program and three months after the conclusion of the program. The standard of acceptability will be the following: 95 percent of the participating physicians will score 100 percent on the post test. Objectives measured by the questionnaire are listed below.

1. The physician will exhibit an increased awareness of the dimensions of the child-abuse problem on a local level by:
   a) identifying reported incidence of figures.
   b) stating the estimated extent of underreporting.
   c) identifying the child-abuse mortality rates.
   d) identifying the percentage of abused children who sustain permanent disabilities as a result of abuse.
2. The physician will demonstrate knowledge of the referral and support systems for child abuse in the community by:
   a) listing three possible resources available in the community for immediate consultation (pediatric social worker, local pediatrician on the hospital staff who has expertise in the management of child abuse cases, and Children's Protective Agency).
   b) identifying three agencies that are available for treatment of child abusers in the community (Parents Anonymous, psychiatric service at the hospital, Department of Social Services at the hospital).
   c) stating the proper sequence of physician activities in initiating a referral for child abuse.
   d) stating the activities and functions of the pediatric social worker and the Children's Protective Agency relevant to the management of abused children.
3. The physician will demonstrate an increased understanding of the New York state child-abuse statutes by:
   a) stating the legal obligations of physicians to report *suspected* cases of child abuse.
   b) identifying the appropriate agency (Children's Protective Agency) to whom all cases of suspected abuse must be reported.
   c) stating that the physician is protected from liability whenever he reports a suspected case of child abuse.

PROPOSAL 3 — GATHERING BASELINE DATA FOR A MATERNAL HEALTH EDUCATION PROGRAM

Proposal 3 applies the principles of PRECEDE to the development of a maternal health-risk profile from which a specific health education program could be

Prepared in 1978 by Joyce Cameron, Angela Deneris, and Margie Freston, University of Utah; material edited for this book and notes omitted.

developed. In the piece that follows, Cameron, Deneris, and Freston present their justification for the project, after which they outline the social, epidemiologic, and behavioral diagnoses.

Rationale for the Program

It has long been known that the incidence of low birth weights is significantly less among women who initiate prenatal care during the first trimester than it. is among women who initiate it later. Women who receive no prenatal care have, by far, the highest incidence of prematurity. In general, the later in the pregnancy the prenatal care is started, the higher the risk of delivering a low-birth-weight infant.

However, the amount and quality of prenatal care are not the only factors contributing to low birth weights. Many other contributing factors, both behavioral and nonbehavioral, are known, chiefly through retrospective studies. Retrospective studies do not reflect the entire scope of the problem, however, because they are based on past events, possibly incomplete data (obtained from existing records), and possibly faulty memories.

Retrospective studies can give direction to epidemiologic studies of a prospective nature. Prospective studies are much stronger because they allow the observation of events and their interplay to be planned. Women can be followed through pregnancy and the different factors implicated in low birth weights monitored. Baseline data can be gathered, and community-wide profiles of predisposing, enabling, and reinforcing factors developed. From these data, various approaches to more effective prenatal educational programs can be devised.

The purpose of this study is to develop such a community-wide profile and to correlate selected health factors in pregnant women with outcome variables associated with low-birth-weight infants. Analysis of the multiple variables that correlate with low birth weights within a given community will permit identification of specific social, behavioral, and vital indicators. Further classifying contributing variables according to whether they are behavioral or nonbehavioral and determining the predisposing, enabling, and reinforcing factors associated with each will suggest appropriate health education programs specific for a given community. A secondary purpose of this study, then, is to devise a means of assessing a community for health education needs related to prenatal care.

Objectives

Basic to this study is the determination of behavioral and nonbehavioral factors affecting pregnant women in the community. Behavioral factors are those over which a woman might have control; nonbehavioral factors are those over which she has no control. Both types can influence pregnancy outcome, but behavioral factors can be influenced by educational and motivational means.

The objectives of this study are to identify the independent variables that correlate significantly with the infant outcome variables of weight, length of gestational age, and behavior. Five variables have been identified: nutrition, stress, personal habits, physical status, and disease process or conditions.

1. Regarding nutritional factors in relation to pregnant Salt Lake County women, this study proposes to:
   a) describe the nutritional status of women.
   b) identify the predisposing, enabling, and reinforcing factors influencing nutritional behavior during pregnancy.
   c) compile a nutritional profile of pregnant women including the following data: maternal height and weight; three-day diet analysis at three points in pregnancy; measure of subcutaneous fat; and use of supplemental vitamins and minerals. A list of predisposing, enabling, and reinforcing factors will also be included.
   d) identify the nutritional factors that significantly correlate with infant outcome.

2. Regarding stress factors in relation to pregnant Salt Lake County women, this study proposes to:
   a) describe the illness-proneness status of pregnant women according to the Utah IVS test.
   b) determine the percentage of women who are within one standard deviation of the mean, between one and two standard deviations of the mean, and above two standard deviations of the mean of the illness-proneness scale of the Utah IVS test.
   c) compile a stress profile of pregnant women based on the Utah IVS test; pregnancy symptoms; the Cornell Psychiatric Index; and the Schedule of Recent Experience. The Schedule of Recent Experience is an indicator of recent life changes that measures social stress, work stress, family stress, financial stress, life-style stress and personal-habit-changes stress.
   d) identify the stress factors that significantly correlate with infant outcome.

3. Regarding personal-habit factors in relation to pregnant Salt Lake County women, this study proposes to:

     a) describe the habits of pregnant women insofar as smoking, alcohol consumption, medication intake, and caffeine ingestion are concerned.

     b) compile a profile of personal habits of pregnant women.

     c) identify the personal habits that significantly correlate with infant outcome.

4. Regarding physical-status factors in relation to pregnant Salt Lake County women, this study proposes to:

     a) detail nonbehavioral indicators of the physical status of pregnant women, including hematocrit, blood pressure, pulse, respiration, temperature, fundic height, fetal heart rate, fetal activity, and urinalysis.

     b) compile a profile of physical status of pregnant women.

     c) identify the nonbehavioral factors that correlate with infant outcome.

5. Regarding disease process or complicating conditions in relation to pregnant Salt Lake County women, this study proposes to:

     a) determine the incidence and prevalence of disease, disease symptoms, and complicating conditions (whether preexisting, coexisting, or specific to pregnancy) by means of systems-review interviews with pregnant subjects.

     b) compile a profile of disease processes and complicating conditions in pregnant women.

     c) identify these symptoms, conditions, or diseases that significantly correlate with infant outcome.

Social Diagnosis

New procedures in the care and treatment of low-birth-weight infants are saving lives. Although the infant death rate has steadily declined, social problems relative to the birth of low-weight infants are significant, including (1) cost to the family and health-care system of prolonged hospitalization; (2) increased family stress; (3) the need for special community programs; and (4) increased incidence of later abuse. Every low-birth-weight infant born presents a crisis to the family and the community.

Epidemiological Diagnosis

Prenatal care   Early prenatal care can offset the medical and social risks associated with low-birth-weight offspring. It has been estimated that approximately 70 percent of the medical complications that can occur during pregnancy can be anticipated as a result of an initial prenatal examination.

Prenatal care can put women in touch with prenatal educational resources as well. The needs of the pregnant population in terms of prenatal education will differ from community to community.

In Utah (in 1975) 5.3 percent of the live births were low weight; nationally 7.4 percent of all live births were low weight. The difference has been attributed to the fact that 80 percent of all Utah women receive early prenatal care, thus ranking Utah second in the nation for such care. Additionally, the number of prenatal visits in Utah for this year was 11.1, compared with 10.0 prenatal visits for the thirty-eight reporting states. The proportion of low-birth-weight babies will generally decrease as the frequency of prenatal visits increases. However, the quantity and quality of prenatal education currently being offered is unknown.

Demographic variables Information obtained nationally from birth certificates indicates that there are large variations in the quality and kind of prenatal care received by mothers of different social and demographic backgrounds. Differences in the time of initiation of prenatal care have been observed for women of various ages, education levels, marital status, and areas of residence. Within each of these groups, less prenatal care was a consistent pattern for black mothers.

In Utah black women had the highest percentage of low-birth-weight infants; white women had the lowest percentage (table C.3A). White infants accounted for 95 percent of the births in Utah.

Maternal age is another variable that contributes to infant birth weight. Nationally, the teenage mother and the mother older than thirty-five have the highest incidence of low-birth-weight infants. This is also true in Utah, where 8.3 percent of the infants born to mothers nineteen years old or younger and 6.5 percent of infants born to mothers thirty-five years old or older are low birth weight (table C.3B).

TABLE C.3A

Percentage of low-birth-weight infants of total births, by race: Utah, 1975

Race	Percentage of births less than 2,500 grams*
White	5.2
Black	13.8
Indian	5.8
Other nonwhite	5.6
All	5.3

*5.47 pounds.

Behavioral Diagnosis

Nonbehavioral factors   Many nonbehavioral factors contribute to the incidence of low-birth-weight infants. Prenatal health-education efforts may affect behavioral factors but have no impact on nonbehavioral factors. Maternal age and race are nonbehavioral factors that we have already identified.

In addition, mothers living at higher altitudes have smaller babies. Smaller mothers deliver smaller infants. Environmental conditions such as toxic substances around the mother's residence or place of employment can also influence pregnancy outcome.

The expectant mother has virtually no control over problems specific to pregnancy, such as Rh incompatability and cervical incompetence. She cannot prevent certain conditions such as heart disease or renal pathology. Viral or bacterial disease can coexist with pregnancy. Multiple gestation is another nonbehavioral factor. These and other problems may contribute to low birth weights.

Behavioral factors   Health behaviors potentially under the control of the mother and identified in the literature as being possibly correlated with low-birth-weight and other infant problems are those related to (1) maternal nutrition; (2) stress; and (3) personal habits such as smoking and ingestion of alcohol, caffeine, medications, and social drugs.

The basic assumption underlying the importance of behavioral factors is that health is a result of the actions of each person twenty-four hours a day, seven days a week. Pregnancy is a period of increased emotional readiness to look at oneself, to learn, and to grow. The willingness of most couples to carry out health behaviors that have potential for building healthy babies is

TABLE C.3B

Live births, by birth weight and age of mother: Utah, 1975

| Age of mother | Number of live births | Birth weight | | | |
| | | Less than 2,500 grams* | | More than 2,500 grams* | |
	Number	Number	Percent	Number	Percent
Total	31,424	1,681	5.3	29,743	94.6
19 years or younger	3,728	311	8.3	3,417	91.6
20–24 years	12,163	651	5.3	11,512	94.6
25–29 years	9,384	408	4.3	8,976	95.6
30–34 years	4,345	193	4.4	4,152	95.5
35 years or older	1,804	118	6.5	1,686	93.4

*5.47 pounds.

evident to health professionals who work closely with such couples. Childbirth and parenting education is being increasingly recognized as a tremendously valuable resource in creating well-informed health consumers who have the knowledge, skills, coping abilities, confidence, and motivation to positively affect their childbearing outcomes.

Community profiles regarding the status, practices, and knowledge of women relative to the three behavioral factors would materially assist healthcare providers and childbirth educators in formulating health education programs in any given community. Information concerning the predisposing, enabling, and reinforcing factors underlying these health behaviors could give additional program direction. Information regarding the effects of these behaviors on the health of infants of a community could also be a powerful motivating influence for expectant mothers.

Predisposing, Enabling, and Reinforcing Factors

Predisposing factors are the motivating qualities of information, attitudes, values, and perceptions that an individual brings to a given situation such as pregnancy. Enabling factors are forces that facilitate the achievement of a designated outcome such as ingestion of a nutritious diet in pregnancy. Reinforcing factors are those forces that strengthen the motivations and actions of an individual. Behavior that indicates support and caring, for example, can reinforce or strengthen the ability and determination to carry out desired health behaviors. An analysis of predisposing, enabling, and reinforcing factors influencing positive nutrition behavior is given, as an example, in table C.3C.

PROPOSAL 4—A COMPREHENSIVE DENTAL HEALTH EDUCATION PROGRAM FOR LOW-INCOME CHILDREN

Social and epidemiologic diagnoses revealed that dental-health problems were especially prevalent and severe among children of low-income families. In this project a dual educational tack is proposed: (1) a "health skills" program for children and (2) a concurrent "health skills" and motivational program for parents. The rationale behind this approach is that parents are a critical but untapped source of educational support for children. What follows is an excerpt of the proposed programs and a brief statement of an administrative diagnosis. (What is referred to in this proposal as Responsive Education

---

Prepared in 1978 by Gene Berry, Kent Sundquist, and Dorothy Thompson, University of Utah; material edited for this book and notes omitted.

TABLE C.3C

Factors influencing nutrition behavior ranked according to importance and changeability

Factors	Importance	Potential for change if needed
Predisposing factors		
Knowledge		
Nutrient needs in pregnancy (recommended daily allowances for pregnant women of given ages)	Medium	High
Food sources of specific nutrients (including "nutrient-dense" foods)	High	High
Effect of nutrients on the fetus	High	High
Preparation of foods to preserve nutrients	High	High
Attitudes		
Self-confidence (sense of ability to care effectively for oneself)	Medium	Medium
Self-worth (value of self as a person worthy of achievement)	High	Medium
Desire for a healthy outcome for self and baby (desire to improve nutritional practices if deficits in needed nutrients are identified)	High	Medium
Values		
Family practices in nutrition	High	Low
Cultural practices in nutrition	High	Low
Perceptions		
Belief that recommended nutrients will actually benefit the fetus and self	High	High
Sense of control over the course and outcome of pregnancy ("what I eat will make a difference")	High	Medium
Enabling factors		
Ability to obtain and pay for food	High	Medium
Availability of food-supplement programs when needed	High	Medium
Cooking and preparation skills	High	High
Living situation in which choices regarding food purchase and preparation are possible	High	Low
Reinforcing factors		
Support of correct food choices by family and friends	High	Medium
Trust in the health-care provider's and childbirth educator's information and suggestions	High	Medium

is part of a nationwide project to provide continuing educational assistance to Head Start children in elementary school.)

Learning Objectives

To give direction to the learning objectives, the predisposing, enabling, and reinforcing factors having to do with each behavioral objective have been identified, classified, and ranked according to importance and changeability. Changeability rankings are shown in tables C.4A and C.4B. The standard of acceptability in meeting the behavioral objectives will be that 60 percent of the children in the "maximum-involvement group" will adopt the practices of brushing and flossing their teeth twice daily and that 60 percent of the parents of these children will see that they visit dentists every ten to twelve months. Based on the analyses reflected in tables C.4A and C.4B and discussion with Responsive Education Program staff and representative parents, learning objectives for the educational program have been developed. These are listed in tables C.4C and C.4D.

Educational Intervention

The target population for study will be students in the Responsive Education Program in Jackson, Washington, Lincoln, and Bennion schools of the Salt Lake City School District. Franklin school, another Responsive Education school, will not be included in the study because a large percentage of the school's students attend the Neighborhood House day-care center, which already provides dental care and dental education for its students.

Parent Education Program

Minimum-involvement group Informed consent for student involvement in the dental education study and the five dental examinations will be obtained from parents by teachers at Washington and Lincoln schools during student registration. The teachers will explain the in-class dental education program to the parents at this time. They will solicit parental support for the students' dental performance at the beginning of the year. Toothbrushes will be given to parents at this time for the students' daily home use.

Maximum-involvement group Informed consent for student involvement in the dental education study and the five dental examinations will be obtained from parents by teachers at Jackson and Bennion schools during student registration. The parents will be given information about a dental health education class for parents to be held in the school within a week and encouraged to attend.

TABLE C.4A

Classification of causes of parents' behavior

Behavioral objective: For the maximum-involvement group, 60 percent of the parents of children in the Responsive Education Program will take their children to a dentist once every ten to twelve months.

| | *Predisposing Factors* | |
Positive attitudes, beliefs, values:	Negative attitudes, beliefs, values:	Changeability
Parents' belief in the importance of dental visits	Low socioeconomic group membership	Low
Parents' belief in the importance of brushing and flossing	Low educational level	Low
	Lack of awareness of early signs of dental need	Medium
	No knowledge of nutrition and relationship to dental health	Medium

| | *Enabling Factors* | |
Positive	Negative	Changeability
Lists of dentists available who take payments from social agencies and Responsive Education Program	High cost of professional dental care	High
	Lack of oral screening and referral in schools	High
	Difficulty in arranging transportation	Medium

| | *Reinforcing Factors* | |
Positive	Negative	Changeability
Parents' effectiveness as models for going to the dentist	Possibly poor parental attitudes toward regular dental visits	Low
	Lack of health personnel to do necessary follow-ups	High

The in-class dental education program will be explained at this time. Toothbrushes will be given to parents for the students' daily home use.

The parent education class and dental examinations performed at school will be explained further in following sections.

Student Education Program

Students in the experimental groups in the four study schools (Washington, Lincoln, Jackson, and Bennion) will be educated regarding the origin of den-

TABLE C.4B

Classification of causes of children's behavior.

Behavioral objective: For the maximum-involvement group, 60 percent of the children will brush and floss their teeth twice a day by May 1980.

Predisposing Factors		
Positive attitudes, beliefs, values:	Negative attitudes, beliefs, values:	Changeability
Parents' belief in importance of oral maintenance	Lack of recognition by children ages five to nine of the value of brushing and flossing	Low

Enabling Factors		
Positive	Negative	Changeability
Tooth brushes, paste, floss, disclosing tablets, and mirrors provided	Lack of effective plaque-removal skills	Low

Reinforcing Factors		
Positive	Negative	Changeability
Parents' effectiveness as reinforcers of child behavior	Parents' display of poor oral-health behavior	Low
	Teachers' possible objection to taking on dental-health curriculum	Medium
Teachers' and teacher assistants' effectiveness as reinforcers of positive oral-health behavior		

tal disease. Students will be taught how to detect plaque by using disclosing tablets and individual dental mirrors. Brushing and flossing will be done in the classroom daily after lunch. The importance of nutrition in dental health will be discussed, including the importance of reducing intake of carbohydrates and refined sugar. Students will be educated regarding regular professional dental care.

The control group The control group will consist of non-Responsive Education classroom students in corresponding grade levels (kindergarten through third grade) in Jackson, Washington, Lincoln, and Bennion schools. Parental consent will be obtained for the five dental examinations to be performed during the school year by the teachers during registration.

The Salt Lake City School District does not currently offer a dental health education program as comprehensive as the proposed classroom education program. This is not expected to change during the proposed study.

TABLE C.4C

Statement of learning objectives for parents

Knowledge: By the end of the program, 90 percent of the parents will know:
   1. the causes of dental disease
   2. the importance of professional dental care
   3. the importance of oral maintenance and plaque removal
   4. the correlation between nutrition and dental health
   5. how to acquire transportation to professional dental care

Beliefs: By the end of the program, 80 percent of the parents will believe:
   1. that the consequences of poor dental care can be dental disease
   2. that regular professional dental care is valuable
   3. that oral maintenance and plaque removal is important
   4. that there is a correlation between nutrition and dental health
   5. that they can acquire their own transportation to a dentist

Skills: By the end of the program, 70 percent of the parents will be able to:
   1. identify possible areas of dental disease with the use of disclosing tablets and dental mirrors
   2. effectively remove plaque by brushing and flossing their teeth
   3. develop nutritional meal plans for their families
   4. identify a dentist for their family
   5. identify a means of transportation to the dentist

We anticipate, therefore, that any differences in dental indices indicated by the examinations performed simultaneously in Responsive Education and control-group students can be attributed to the proposed dental health education program.

Although topical application of fluoride is known to be an effective agent in dental disease, particularly in nonfluoridated water supply areas such as Utah, it will not be used in this study with the target students. It is hoped that after the completion of the study, it will be possible to gain parental consent to introduce the topical use of fluoride to Responsive Education students.

Staff development   Because teachers are a known reinforcing force in child health education, in-service training for teachers and other program staff will be provided prior to the parent and classroom education program. The training will focus on the importance of dental education and the origin of dental disease and include instruction in techniques of plaque removal.

TABLE C.4D
Statement of learning objectives for children

Knowledge: By the end of the program, 90 percent of the children will know:
1. the value of preventive oral hygiene in preventing dental disease
2. the value of regular professional dental care
3. how to brush and floss their teeth
4. the value of a well-balanced diet and appropriate snacks in promoting good dental health

Beliefs: By the end of the program, 80 percent of the children will believe:
1. that daily brushing and flossing combined with regular professional dental care will prevent dental disease
2. that a well-balanced diet and appropriate snacks will improve dental health

Skills: By the end of the program, 70 percent of the children will be able to:
1. brush and floss their teeth properly
2. understand and use disclosing tablets and dental mirrors
3. choose foods and snacks that are appropriate to maintaining good dental health

Educational Strategies

Maximum-involvement group: Parents The strategies to be used in the proposed parent education program are lecture, individual instruction, small-group discussion, audiovisual aids, programmed learning, and modeling. This variety of strategies was selected because of the characteristics of the target parent population: The parents are educationally disadvantaged, and their social milieu is noncohesive and poorly integrated. The group is heterogeneous, with most members of low socioeconomic status. Their motivation is weak, and they have little idea of the severity of dental disease or of their susceptibility to it. Social acceptability of the desired behavior is high; however, adherence to the therapeutic regimen is expected to be poor.

The educational strategies will be used during three class periods of two hours each to be held during consecutive weeks. The class will be conducted by the program nurse and dental hygienist. The strategies will also be used in subsequent follow-up maximum-involvement group contacts.

During the first class, the origin of dental disease will be discussed. Parents will be trained to use disclosing tablets and dental mirrors to detect plaque. Through individual instruction and role modeling parents will be trained in brushing and flossing skills. Toothbrushes will be supplied for use by students and parents at home. Parents will also take home disclosing tablets and dental mirrors, with the recommendation that they be used weekly, biweekly, and then monthly as family plaque-removal skills improve.

During the second class, information on the origin of dental disease will be reviewed, as will techniques of plaque detection and removal. The importance of nutrition and the reduction of intake of refined sugar will be introduced using lecture, small-group discussion, and audiovisual methods. Individual family diets will be analyzed, and recommendations for changes provided.

During the third class, information on the origin of dental disease will again be reviewed. This review will be accompanied by further discussion of the importance of reducing intake of refined sugar and discussion of family efforts at plaque detection and removal and dietary changes for the preceding weeks. An additional subject for discussion during this class will be transportation and communication problems parents might have in acquiring professional dental care. Each class member will identify a dentist to be used by his or her family and a method for contacting the dentist and means of transportation to be used. Each class member will determine dates for necessary dental examinations for all members of his or her family and make a record for future use.

Throughout the program study year, Responsive Education Program monthly newsletters will be used as a source for additional dental health information to all Responsive Education Program parents. Basic dental health education will be included.

Students in the maximum-involvement group will be evaluated for "high dental risk" characteristics using the dental-evaluation indices performed at school. Parents of "high dental risk" students, that is, students with high scores on the indices, will be contacted by the program nurse or dental hygienist and the indices scores discussed. If the parent attended the parent education class, arrangements for a home visit by the nurse or dental hygienist will be made. During the home visit, principles discussed in classes will be reviewed, as will plaque-removal skills. If the parent did not attend the parent education classes, arrangements for a home visit or visits by the nurse or dental hygienist will be made, and the pertinent information and techniques provided.

Maximum-involvement group: Students   The strategies to be used throughout the proposed classroom program are lecture, individual instruction, small-group discussion, simulation and games, audiovisual aids, programmed learning, educational television, and modeling. This variety of strategies was selected because of the unique characteristics of the target population, namely, age (kindergarten through third grades), educational status (disadvantaged), social noncohesiveness, poor integration, and heterogeneity. The children, predominantly of low socioeconomic status, are weakly motivated and have little understanding of the potential severity of dental disease and their susceptibility to it. Social acceptability of the behavior to be learned is high; however, as with the parents, adherence to the therapeutic regimen is expected to be poor.

The classroom educational strategies will be used after the initial evaluation has provided baseline data. Brushing and flossing will be done daily, accompanied by weekly, biweekly, and, later, monthly use of disclosing tablets and dental mirrors to indicate effectiveness of plaque removal. Students with evident problems will receive individual attention from the dental hygienist, nurse, or teacher. The dental hygienist will evaluate the dental health of children in both the control and study groups at five separate times during the period of the study using plaque and gingival indices. Results of the evaluations will be mailed to the parents of children in both groups.

Administrative Diagnosis

One of the major barriers to the success of this study could be lack of cooperation from the school district. However, the free dental checks offered throughout the year to children in the control group will require minimal effort on the part of classroom teachers and school principals. This, coupled with the fact that the Responsive Education nurse, teachers, and administration are supportive of the project, should make it less difficult to gain the support of the school district administration.

Whether or not we can establish the parents in the maximum-involvement group as reinforcers of the children's dental-health behaviors by getting them to the dental education classes and maintaining their willingness to practice good dental health at home throughout the year is also a concern. Fortunately, the Responsive Education staff, parent coordinators, and teachers already have established positive working relationships with the parents, and their attitudes toward parental involvement are positive. We feel that this situation will facilitate the delivery of the dental program to the children and their parents. In addition, the parent coordinators of the Responsive Education Program currently maintain personal contact with program parents and will continue to do so during the period of the study.

Funding of the program will eliminate the barriers associated with insufficient personnel and materials and the parents' inability to pay for professional dental care for their children. These have traditionally been barriers to effective dental education.

1. P. E. Enterline, "Pitfalls in Epidemiologic Research: An Examination of the Asbestos Literature," *Journal of Occupational Medicine* 18 (1976) 150–56; J. W. Lloyd, "Long-Term Mortality Study of Steelworkers. V. Respiratory Cancer in Coke-Plant Workers," *Journal of Occupational Medicine* 13 (1971): 53–66.

Suggested Criteria and Rating Scales for Evaluation of Structure and Process

SOME SUGGESTED CRITERIA FOR EVALUATION OF PROGRAMME STRUCTURE AND PROCESS

A. Problem diagnosis stage

1. Data from available sources (e.g. health department, school district, etc.) should have been gathered and consolidated for planning purposes (data on both the problem and the population).
2. Existing literature on specific problem or population should have been reviewed prior to planning.
3. Available resources should have been surveyed in the community to avoid overlap and to identify individuals and groups with prior experience with the problem.

Reprinted from Lawrence W. Green et al., *Guidelines for Health Education in Maternal and Child Health, International Journal of Health Education* 21 (supplement), no. 3 (July–September 1978): 1–33, by permission of the editor and senior author.

    4. Consultation with health authorities at national or regional level should have been utilized where specific data, literature, resources or experience are lacking.

B. *Planning stage*
    1. The specific target and transmitter populations should have been identified (geographic, ethnic, SES, age, etc.).
    2. Representatives from the "target" and transmitter population should have been included from the beginning of the formal planning.
    3. Representatives from each level and occupational category ultimately responsible for implementing the programme should have been included in the planning.
    4. Objectives for the programme should have been stated from the consumer's perspective, i.e. in terms of *their* goals and with numerical targets.
    5. Priorities should have been established among objectives.
    6. Participating agencies should have been represented throughout the planning.
    7. Participating personnel within each agency should have been kept informed of progress on planning.
    8. Planning sessions should have been varied in format and location to provide opportunities for input from individuals and groups who are more or less responsive under different circumstances.
    9. Planning should not have ended with submittal of the grant proposal or receipt of the contract or budget.
    10. As much attention should have been given to the knowledge, attitudes, values and social relationships of the target population as to their behaviour.
    11. The community at large should have been kept informed of developments at all stages of the programme.

C. *Preparation stage*
    1. Specific programme and service components should have been specified (e.g. what kind of prevention, training or treatment).
    2. All participating staff should have received a full orientation to the programme objectives, philosophy, and limitations.
    3. Volunteers should have been recruited and existing staff with major responsibilities in the programme should have been provided in-service training to assume their new roles in the programme.
    4. Supervisory responsibilities should have been clearly delineated.
    5. Specific staff functions should have been clearly delineated.

6. Specific audio or visual aides collected or produced for the programme should have been carefully pretested in the populations with which they are to be used.
7. Opinion leaders in the community who may not have been directly involved in the early planning should have been involved at this stage to preclude their opposition during implementation of the programme.
8. Commitments on personnel, physical facilities, financial assets and supplies should have been reasonably firm before implementing programme.
9. Evaluation design and sampling should have been developed.
10. All record-keeping forms for service data in the programme should have been developed and pretested.
11. Referral sources and cooperating agencies should have been lined up and informed of beginning date for the programme.
12. Methods of recruiting consumers should have been specified.

D. *Implementation stage*
1. Publicity spread or promotion of the services should have been limited at first to avoid creating more demand for services than can adequately be met at the outset.
2. High priority cases or groups should have been handled first. Satisfied clients should have been a major goal of the initial services rendered.
3. Data collection and record-keeping procedures should have been appropriately applied and monitored.
4. Criteria specific to film or videotape showing
   a) Films should have been previewed several days in advance of their scheduled showing, with representatives of target audience reacting to preview.
   b) Audiences should have been small enough and homogeneous enough to allow intimate discussion following film showings.
   c) Verbal introduction of film should have included a statement on the purpose of showing the film, reasons for selecting it, what to look for and what aspects will be discussed following the film.
5. Criteria specific to professional training workshops
   a) A normative ratio of cost per teacher-day of training provided should have been developed and used as one index of programme support.
   b) The programme should have had the active support of school administrators, teacher's union (if any), and parent-teacher associations, or professional association.

c) Teachers should have been allowed release time (with pay) or received graduate credit (where such exists) or both.

6. Staff and supervisors should have performed the functions specified (C 4 & 5 above).
7. Programme should have made appropriate use of volunteers, audio and visual aides, cooperating agencies and referral sources (C 3, 6, 7 and 11 above).
8. Communication and feedback should have been maintained between personnel at all programme levels (vertical) and between cooperating agencies or groups (horizontal).

SUGGESTED RATING SCALES ON CRITERIA OF PROGRAMME STRUCTURE AND PROCESS

A. Problem diagnosis stage

1. Scale 0 = Little or no attempt to collect data on problem or population.

    1 = Some attempt to collect, but no attempt to consolidate or use data; or data collected on population but not on problem, or on problem but not on population.

    2 = Reasonable efforts to collect and consolidate data from available sources on both population characteristics and problems.

2. Scale 0 = No evidence of serious review of scientific literature on the problem prior to planning.

    1 = Some evidence of literature review prior to planning but not recorded or used in the planning; or literature systematically reviewed on population but not on problem, or on problem but not on population.

    2 = Clear documentation of previous research and experience pertinent to the problem and population.

3. Scale 0 = No effort to interview other agency representatives in the community who may have had prior experience with the problem.

    1 = Some effort to interview others, but some obvious omissions, or some clearly wasteful overlap in services.

    2 = Rather thorough survey of available resources and individuals having had prior experience with the problem in the community.

4. Scale 0 = No effort to consult national or regional officials where specific data, literature, resources or experience were lacking.

    1 = Some assistance or consultation obtained but not actively sought or not obtained until after the planning stage.

    2 = Consultation used where specific data, literature, resources or experience were lacking.

B. *Planning stage*

1. Scale 0 = No clear understanding or agreement on whom the programme is intended to serve or who is to transmit the programme.

    1 = Agreement on some but not all of the following: geographic boundaries, ethnic groups, socio-economic groups and age groups to be served.

    2 = Written identification of specific target groups and transmitter groups.

2. Scale 0 = No representatives from the target and transmitter populations actively included in the planning.

    1 = Nominal representation of target population and/or transmitters in planning but not in sufficient numbers or positions to affect decisions: or too late in the planning; or their suggestions ignored or discarded.

    2 = Adequate, active and early participation of representatives of the target and transmitter populations.

3. Scale 0 = No representation of "staff" at any but top levels in planning.

    1 = Representation from middle levels of staff but not from lower levels, or only token participation of lower levels.

    2 = Adequate, active and early participation of representatives from all levels of staff.

4. Scale 0 = No objectives explicitly stated for programme.

    1 = Objectives stated entirely from the perspective of the agency, or in very vague terms.

    2 = Objectives stated in concrete, numerical terms and in terms of target population's goals.

5. Scale 0 = Objectives have no implicit priority (or no objectives stated).

    1 = Objectives have no explicit priority ranking.

2 = Objectives are explicitly ranked according to agreed-upon priorities.

6. Scale 0 = No representation of participating agencies in planning.

1 = Nominal participation only.

2 = Adequate, active and early participation of affiliating agencies throughout the planning.

7. Scale 0 = No attempt to inform personnel until after plans were complete.

1 = Only middle and top level personnel kept informed during planning.

2 = All personnel kept fully informed throughout the planning.

8. Scale 0 = All planning sessions held in one place, most convenient to originator and less to others.

1 = Planning sessions held in two locations, but format always same with originator as chairman.

2 = Planning sessions varied in location and format to elicit input from different groups who are more or less responsive under different circumstances.

9. Scale 0 = Planning consisted of one meeting prior to submittal of grant proposal, contract bid or budget.

1 = Planning consisted of more than one meeting but ended with receipt of grant, contract or budget.

2 = Planning continued with participation after receipt of grant, contract or budget.

10. Scale 0 = Planning based exclusively on behavior of the "target" groups.

1 = Planning based on presumed knowledge, attitudes, values and social relationships of the target populations.

2 = Planning based on concrete data concerning knowledge, attitudes, values and social relationships of target groups.

11. Scale 0 = Programme plan announced to the community at large only after programme was underway.

1 = Programme plan announced to the community after grant, contract or budget was received.

2 = Programme idea announced to community before planning was far advanced and community kept informed of progress on planning.

C. Preparation stage

1. Scale 0 = No specification of programme and service components beyond general programme objectives.

   1 = Services itemized but not clearly related to programme objectives.

   2 = Programme and service components clearly delineated and related to programme objectives.

2. Scale 0 = Staff assigned duties without any orientation to overall programme objectives, philosophy and limitations.

   1 = Staff assigned duties with minimal written orientation material.

   2 = Staff involved in mutual orientation programme at which responsibilities and functions were assigned within the context of programme objectives, philosophy, service components and limitations.

3. Scale 0 = No recruitment or training of staff or volunteers before programme services began.

   1 = Recruitment of staff and/or volunteers before programme initiated, but no training.

   2 = Recruitment and training of staff and volunteers preceded programme services.

4. Scale 0 = No clear designation of organizational hierarchy or lines of authority.

   1 = Hierarchy designated by an organization chart, but no clear indication of supervisory responsibilities.

   2 = Supervisory responsibilities clearly delineated at each level of organization.

5. Scale 0 = Specific staff functions not indicated beyond programme objectives.

   1 = Job descriptions include specific responsibilities, but not related to programme objectives or service components.

   2 = Staff functions clearly delineated in relation to programme objectives.

6. Scale 0 = Audiovisual aides not pretested.

   1 = Audiovisual aides pretested with staff or others not in the "target" population.

   2 = Audiovisual aides pretested in the "target" population.

7. Scale 0 = Opposition encountered from community opinion

leaders who could have been, but were not, included in planning or preparation.

1 = No opposition encountered but some anticipated from community leaders still not involved in the programme.

2 = Efforts made to involve community opinion leaders in the preparation stage who were not involved in earlier planning.

8. Scale 0 = Programme initiated with few or no commitments firm on personnel, physical facilities, financial assets and supplies.

1 = Programme delayed because commitments were not lined up sufficiently in advance of planned implementation date.

2 = Personnel, facilities, budget, equipment and supplies lined up in advance of planned implementation date.

9. Scale 0 = Evaluation given no formal consideration prior to implementation of the programme.

1 = Evaluation considered during planning and preparation but no written plan or design.

2 = Evaluation design and sampling plan well developed prior to implementation of the programme.

10. Scale 0 = No record-keeping forms for service data developed prior to initiation of services.

1 = Record-keeping forms developed but not pretested prior to initiation of services.

2 = Record-keeping forms well developed and pretested prior to initiation of programme services.

11. Scale 0 = No referral sources officially contacted prior to programme initiation.

1 = Referral sources contacted but not prepared to provide or receive referrals at time of programme opening.

2 = Referral sources providing and/or receiving referrals at time of opening of programme.

12. Scale 0 = No specific plan for recruitment of consumers or users of services at time services began.

1 = Recruitment plans limited to mass media announcements.

2 = Well developed outreach plans to recruit specific target groups according to priorities dictated by objectives.

D. *Implementation stage*

1 and

2. Scale 0 = Initial publicity or promotion of services directed more to low priority target groups than to high priority groups.

     1 = Initial promotion of services spread equally without regard to priority groups or to limitations of services.

     2 = Initial promotion efforts directed primarily at high priority groups and without creating more demand for services that can adequately be met at the outset.

3. Scale 0 = No records kept during initial services.

     1 = Records kept but not according to plans or not appropriate to objectives.

     2 = Records kept according to plans and objectives.

4. Scale 0 = Audiences for film showings too large (over 20) and heterogeneous for intimate discussion following showings.

     1 = Audiences homogeneous but too large; or small enough but too mixed to obtain intimate discussion.

     2 = Audiences small enough and homogeneous enough to allow intimate discussion of films.

5. Scale 0 = Films used without introduction.

     1 = Film showings preceded by introductions but not followed by discussion, or introduction not related to discussion.

     2 = Verbal introduction of films included a statement on the purpose of showing the film, reasons for selecting it, what to look for and what aspects will be discussed following the film.

6. Scale 0 = Staff and supervisors not in positions specified by plan.

     1 = Staff in appropriate positions but not performing functions specified by plan.

     2 = Staff and supervisors performing functions specified by programme plan.

7. Scale 0 = Volunteers, audio and visual aides, cooperating agencies and referral sources not being used in programme.

     1 = Resources being used but not according to plans.

     2 = Resources being appropriately used according to plan (or plan appropriately and officially adjusted to fit resources).

8. Scale 0 = Neither vertical communication between staff nor horizontal communication with other agencies is satisfactory.

1 = Communication and feedback adequate within the organization but not with cooperating agencies, or vice versa.

2 = Communication and feedback maintained within and between cooperating agencies or groups.

Notes

CHAPTER 1

1. M. Mueller, "HMO Act of 1973," Social Security Administration, Office of Research and Statistics, Note no. 5, 1974, quoted in *Medical Care Review,* April 1974, p. 704.

2. *Focal Points,* Bureau of Health Education, DHEW, July 1977.

3. Ibid., September 1976.

4. L. Levin, A. Katz, and E. Holst, *Self Care: Lay Initiatives in Health* (New York: Prodist, 1976); K. Sehnert, *How to Be Your Own Doctor Sometimes* (New York: Grosset & Dunlap, 1975).

5. M. LaLonde, *A New Perspective on the Health of Canadians* (Ottawa, Canada: Ministry of National Health and Welfare, 1974).

6. H. Schnocks, "Foreword," in *Health Education in Europe,* 2d ed., eds. A. Kaplan and R. Erben (Geneva: *International Journal of Health Education,* 1976), p. v.

7. Ibid., p. 209.

8. J. W. Farquhar et al., "Community Education for Cardiovascular Health," *Lancet* 1, no. 8023 (June 4, 1977): 1192–95; L. W. Green, D. M. Levine, and S. G. Deeds, "Clinical Trials of Health Education for Hypertensive Outpatients: Design and Baseline Data," *Preventive Medicine* 4 (1975): 417–25; L. W. Green et al., *The Dacca Family Planning Experiment: A Comparative Evaluation of Programs Directed at Males and at Females,* Pacific Health Education Reports, no. 3 (Berkeley: University of California Press, 1972); H. A. K. Kanaaneh et al., "The Eradication of a Large Scabies Outbreak Using Community-wide Health Education, *American Journal of Public Health* 66 (June 1976): 564–67; T. Drummond, *Using the Method of Paulo Freire in Nutrition Education: An Experimental Plan for Community Action in Northeast Brazil,* Cornell International Nutrition Monograph Series, no. 3 (Ithaca, N.Y.: Cornell University Press, 1975); B. Tomic et al., "A Community Conquers Health," *International Health Education* 20, supplement no. 2 (April–June 1977); P. M. Lazes et al., "Improving Patient Care Through Participation: The Newark Experiment in Staff and Patient Involvement," *International Journal of Health Education* 20 (1977): 61–68.

9. *Report of the President's Committee on Health Education* (New York: Public Affairs Institute, 1973).

10. E. M. Sliepcevich, "Impressions of an Overviewer," in *Proceedings: Preparation and Practice of Community, Patient and School Health Educators,* DHEW, Bureau of Health Manpower (1978), p. 16.

11. D. N. Richards, "Methods and Effectiveness of Health Education: The Past, Present and Future of Social Scientific Involvement," *Social Science and Medicine* 9 (1975), p. 151.

12. J. Knowles, "The Responsibility of the Individual," *Daedalus* 106 (Winter 1977), p. 60.

13. I. M. Rosenstock, "General Criteria for Evaluating Health Education Programs," in *Proceedings of the National Heart and Lung Institute Working Conference on Health Behavior,* DHEW pub. no. (NIH) 76-868 (1975), p. 141.

14. S. Polgar, "Health Actions in Cross-cultural Perspective," in *Handbook of Medical Sociology,* eds. H. E. Freeman, S. Levine, and L. G. Reeder (Englewood Cliffs, N.J.: Prentice-Hall, 1963).

15. A. J. Chwalow, "Contact vs. Content: The Effect of the Multiplicity of Health Education Encounters on Compliance and Blood Pressure Control" (Dr.P.H. diss., Johns Hopkins University School of Hygiene and Public Health, 1978); V. L. Wang, P. Ephross, and L. W. Green, "The Point of Diminishing Returns in Nutrition Education Through Home Visits by Aides: An Evaluation of EFNEP," *Health Education Monographs* 3 (Spring 1975): 70–88.

16. S. G. Deeds, *A Guidebook for Family Planning Education,* DHEW pub. no. (HSA) 74-16002, Bureau of Community Health Services, (1973).

17. M. Minkler, "The Use of Incentives in Family Planning Programmes," *International Journal of Health Education* 19, supplement no. 3 (1976).

18. A. E. Kazdin, *Behavior Modification in Applied Settings* (Homewood, Ill.: Dorsey, 1975).

19. E. Ubell, "Health Behavior Change: A Political Model," *Preventive Medicine* 1 (1972): 209–21.

20. M. J. Mahoney, *Cognitive Behavior Modification* (New York: Balinger, 1977).

21. C. E. Thoresen and M. J. Mahoney, *Self-Control: Power to the Person* (Monterey, Calif.: Brooks/Cole, 1974); L. W. Green et al., "Research and Demonstration Issues in Self-care: Measuring the Decline of Medicocentrism," *Health Education Monographs* 5 (Summer 1977): 161–89.

22. E. M. Rogers, *Communication of Innovations: A Cross-Cultural Approach* (New York: Free Press, 1971).

23. E. M. Rogers, *Communication Strategies for Family Planning* (New York, Free Press, 1973); P. R. Mico and H. S. Ross, *Health Education and Behavioral Science* (Oakland: Third Party, 1975); L. W. Green, "Diffusion and Adoption of Innovations Related to Cardiovascular Risk Behavior in the Public," in *Applying Behavioral Sciences to Cardiovascular Risk,* eds. A. Enelow and J. B. Henderson (New York: American Heart Association, 1975).

24. L. W. Green, "Should Health Education Abandon Attitude Change Strategies? Perspectives from Recent Research," *Health Education Monographs* 1, no. 30 (1970): 25–48.

25. Sliepcevich, "Impressions of an Overviewer"; Thoresen and Mahoney, *Self-Control;* L. Maiman, L. W. Green, and G. Gibson, "Educational Self-treatment by Adult Asthmatics," *Journal of the American Medical Association,* 241 (May 4, 1979): 1919–22. D. L. Roter, "Patient Participation in the Patient-Provider Interaction: The Effects of Patient Question-Asking on the Quality of Interaction, Satisfaction and Compliance," *Health Education Monographs* 5 (Winter 1977): 281–315.

26. Health Education Center, *Strategies for Health Education in Local Health Departments* (Baltimore: Maryland State Department of Health and Mental Hygiene, 1977).

27. L. W. Green et al., *Guidelines for Health Education in Maternal and Child Health, International Journal of Health Education* 21 (supplement), no. 3 (July–September 1978): 1–33.

28. N. Danforth and B. Swaboda, *Agency for International Development Health Education Study* (Washington, D.C.: Westinghouse Health Systems, March 17, 1978).

29. A. Ackerman and H. Kalmer, "Health Education and a Baccalaureate Nursing Curriculum—Myth or Reality (Paper presented at the 105th annual meeting of the American Public Health Association, Washington, D.C., November 1, 1977).

30. D. Fedder and R. Beardsley, "Training Pharmacists to Become Patient Educators" (Paper presented to the section of teachers of pharmacy administration of the annual meeting of the American Association of Colleges of Pharmacy, Orlando, Florida, July 18, 1978).

31. B. I. Bennett, "A Model for Teaching Health Education Skills to Primary Care Practitioners," *International Journal of Health Education* 20, no. 4 (1977): 232–39.

32. N. Milio, "A Framework for Prevention: Changing Health-Damaging to Health-Generating Life Patterns," *American Journal of Public Health* 66 (May 1976): 435–39; V. Navarro, *Medicine Under Capitalism* (New York: Prodist, 1976).

33. R. Andersen, *A Behavioral Model of Families' Use of Health Services,* University of Chicago Center for Health Administration Studies Research Series, no. 25 (Chicago: University of Chicago Press, 1968).

34. M. H. Becker, ed., *The Health Belief Model and Personal Health Behavior, Health Education Monographs* 2 (Winter 1974): 324–508.

CHAPTER 2

1. R. R. Faden and A. I. Faden, *Ethical Issues in Public Health Policy: Health Education and Lifestyle Interventions, Health Education Monographs* 6, no. 2 (Summer 1978).
2. L. W. Green, "Toward Cost-Benefit Evaluations of Health Education: Some Concepts, Methods and Examples," ibid. 2, supplement no. 1 (1974): 34–64.
3. Idem, "Determining the Impact and Effectiveness of Health Education As It Relates to Federal Policy," ibid. 6, supplement no. 1 (1978): 28–66.
4. J. L. Dallas, "Health Education: Enabler for a Higher Quality of Life," *Health Services Reports* 87, no. 10 (December 1972): 910–18; C. N. D'Onofrio, "SOPHE and the Quality of Life," ibid.: 955–57.
5. N. Bradburn and D. Capolvitz, *Reports on Happiness: A Pilot Study of Behavior Related to Mental Health* (New York: Aldine, 1965); A. Campbell, P. E. Converse, and W. L. Rodgers, *The Quality of American Life: Perceptions, Evaluations and Satisfactions* (New York: Russell Sage, 1976); K. T. Chun, S. Cobb, and J. R. P. French, Jr., *Measures for Psychological Assessment: A Guide to 3,000 Original Sources and Their Applications* (Ann Arbor: University of Michigan Institute for Social Research, 1975); C. Eastman, A. Randall, and P. L. Hoffer, "How Much to Abate Pollution?," *Public Opinion Quarterly* 38 (Winter 1974–75): 574–84; M. O. Finkelstein, P. A. Pickerel, and G. J. Glasser, "The Death of Children: A Nonparametric Statistical Analysis of Compensation for Anguish," *Columbia Law Review* 74 (June 1974): 884–93; D. W. Fischer, "On the Problems of Measuring Environmental Benefits and Costs," *Social Science Information* 13 (April 1974): 95–105; M. W. Kreuter and L. W. Green, "Evaluation of School Health Education: Identifying Purpose, Keeping Perspective," *Journal of School Health* 48 (April 1978): 228–35; H. Mersky, "Assessment of Pain," *Physiotherapy* 60 (April 1974): 96–98; Environmental Protection Agency, *The Quality of Life Concept: A Potential Tool for Decision-Makers* (March 1973); V. L. Wang, "Social Goals, Health Policy and the Dynamics of Development As Bases for Health Education," *International Journal of Health Education* 20 (1977): 13–18.
6. Wang, "Social Goals, Health Policy and Dynamics of Development"; C. I. Anderson, R. Morton, and L. W. Green, *Community Health*, 3d ed. (St. Louis: Mosby, 1978).
7. Environmental Protection Agency, *Quality of Life Concept*, p. 11–49.
8. G. J. Warheit, R. A. Bell, and J. J. Schwab, *Needs Assessment Approaches: Concepts and Methods*, DHEW pub. no. (ADM) 77-472 National Institute of Mental Health, (1977).
9. Bradburn and Capolvitz, *Reports on Happiness*.
10. R. Needle and K. Swawlewitz, "A Study of Work and the Workplace: Implications of the Psychosocial Aspects for Health Education and an Occupational Health and Safety Program on a University Campus" (Paper presented at the annual meeting of the American College Health Association, New Orleans, 1978).

11. A. H. Van de Ven and A. L. Delbecq, "The Nominal Group As a Research Instrument for Exploratory Health Studies," *American Journal of Public Health* 62 (March 1972): 337–42; W. L. Blockstein, A. R. Bailey, and R. H. Hansen, "Expanding the Role of a University in Consumer Health Education," *Health Education Monographs* 3 (Spring 1975): 62–69; A. L. Delbecq, A. H. Van de Ven, and D. A. Gustafson, *Group Techniques for Program Planning* (Glenview, Ill.: Scott, Foresman, 1975).

12. Van de Ven and Delbecq, "The Nominal Group As a Research Instrument."

13. G. D. Gilmore, "Needs Assessment Processes for Community Health Education," *International Journal of Health Education* 20 (1977): 164–73.

14. Ibid.

15. J. E. Fletcher and H. B. Thompson, "On the Problems of Measuring Environmental Benefits and Costs," *Social Science Information* 13 (April 1974): 95–105; A. S. Linsky, "Stimulating Responses to Mailed Questionnaires: A Review," *Public Opinion Quarterly* 39 (Spring 1975): 82–101.

16. G. T. Dalis and B. B. Strasser, *Teaching Strategies for Values Awareness and Decision Making in Health Education* (Thorofare, N.J.: Slack, 1977).

17. M. Kreuter, "An Interaction Model to Facilitate Awareness and Behavior Change," *Journal of School Health* 46 (November 1976): 543–45; idem, "Health Activation: Personal Responsibility in Prevention," *Proceedings of the 12th Annual Prospective Medicine Conference* (San Diego: Society for Prospective Medicine, 1977).

18. R. E. Berry, Jr., and J. P. Boland, *The Economic Cost of Alcohol Abuse and Alcoholism* (Boston: Policy Analysis, 1974).

19. M. L. C. Bowman, "Assessing College Student Attitudes Toward Environmental Issues," *Journal of Environmental Education* 6 (Winter 1974): 1–5; F. S. Jaffe, "Short-term Costs and Benefits of United States Family Planning Programs," *Studies in Family Planning* 5 (March 1974): 98–105.

20. A. Fonoroff and L. Levin, eds., "Issues in Self-Care," *Health Education Monographs* 5 (Summer 1977): 108–89.

21. Wang, "Social Goals, Health Policy and Dynamics of Development."

22. Green, "Toward Cost-Benefit Evaluations of Health Education"; idem, "Determining Impact and Effectiveness of Health Education."

23. R. Reinhart and J. Cazavelan, "Mental Health Consumer Survey on a Shoestring Budget—It Is Possible!," *American Journal of Community Psychology* 3 (September 1975): 273–76.

24. Warheit, Bell, and Schwab, *Needs Assessment Approaches.*

CHAPTER 3

1. N. Milio, *The Care of Health in Communities: Access for Outcasts* (New York: Macmillan, 1975); National Center for Health Statistics, *Infant Mortality Rates: Socioeconomic Factors, U.S.,* DHEW, March 1972; J. Kosa, A. Antonovsky, and I. K. Zola, eds., *Poverty and Health: A Sociological Analysis* (Cambridge, Mass.: Harvard University Press, 1969).

2. L. W. Green et al., "Guidelines for Health Education in Maternal and Child Health," *International Journal of Health Education* 21 (supplement), no. 3 (July–September 1978): 1–33.

3. *Baselines for Setting Health Goals and Standards,* DHEW pub. no. (HRA) 77-640 Health Resources Administration (1977).

4. M. Lalonde, *A New Perspective on the Health of Canadians* (Ottawa, Canada: Ministry of National Health and Welfare, 1974).

5. Hypertension Detection and Follow-Up Program Cooperation Group, "Race, Education and Prevalence of Hypertension." *American Journal of Epidemiology* 106 (1971): 351–61.

6. National Center for Health Statistics, *Blood Pressure of Persons 6–74 Years of Age in the United States,* NCHS Advance Data no. 1 (October 18, 1976).

7. A. H. Abudejaja, "Some Determinants of Compliance with Treatment Following Blood Pressure Screening" (Ph.D. diss., Johns Hopkins University School of Hygiene and Public Health, 1978).

8. L. W. Green, "Determining the Impact and Effectiveness of Health Education As It Relates to Federal Policy," *Health Education Monographs* 6, supplement no. 1 (1978): 28–66.

9. *Forward Plan for Health FY 1977–81,* DHEW pub. no. (OS) 76-50024 Public Health Service (August 1975).

10. Green, "Determining the Impact and Effectiveness of Health Education As It Relates to Federal Policy."

11. Abudejaja, "Determinants of Compliance with Treatment."

CHAPTER 4

1. L. W. Green, "Quality in Patient Education. What Is It and How Do We Measure It?," in *National Symposium on Patient Education, September 24–26, 1977, Proceedings* (Atlanta: Bureau of Health Education, Center for Disease Control, 1978).

2. A. Rogers-Warren and S. F. Warren, *Ecological Perspectives in Behavior Analysis* (Baltimore: University Park, 1977).

3. H. Selye, *The Stress of Life* (New York: McGraw-Hill, 1956); M. Friedman and R. Rosenman, *Type A Behavior and Your Heart* (New York: Knopf, 1974); C. D. Jenkins, "Components of the Coronary-prone Behavior Pattern—New Relations to Silent Myocardial Infarction and Blood Lipids," *Journal of Chronic Disease* 19 (1966): 599–609.

4. E. M. Rogers and F. F. Shoemaker, *Communication of Innovations: A Cross-Cultural Approach,* 2d ed. (New York: Free Press, 1971).

5. Ibid.; A. L. McAlister et al., "Behavioral Science Applied to Cardiovascular Health: Progress and Research Needs in the Modification of Risk-taking Habits in Adult Populations," *Health Education Monographs* 4 (Spring 1976): 45–74.

6. N. O. Borhani, "Primary Prevention of Coronary Heart Disease: A Critique," *American Journal of Cardiology* 40 (August 1977), p. 258.

CHAPTER 5

1. S. Croog and N. Peters, "Health Beliefs and Smoking; Patterns in Heart Patients and Their Wives: A Longitudinal Study," *American Journal of Public Health* 67 (October 1977), p. 922.

2. D. Cartwright, "Some Principles of Mass Persuasion: Selected Findings from Research on the Sale of United States War Bonds," *Human Relations* 2 (1949): 253–69.

3. J. W. Farquhar et al., "Community Education for Cardiovascular Health," *Lancet* 1, no. 8023 (June 4, 1977): 1192–95.

4. I. M. Rosenstock, "Historical Origins of the Health Belief Model," *Health Education Monographs* 2 (1974): 328–35.

5. H. Kelman, "Attitudes Are Alive and Well and Gainfully Employed in the Sphere of Action," *American Psychologist* 29 (May 1974): 310–24.

6. G. M. Hochbaum, *Public Participation in Medical Screening Programs: A Socio-Psychological Study,* Public Health Service pub. no. 572 (1959); I. M. Rosenstock, "Why People Use Health Services," *Milbank Memorial Fund Quarterly* 44 (July 1966): 94–127; H. Leventhal and R. P. Singer, "Affect Arousal and Positioning of Recommendations in Persuasive Communications," *Journal of Personality and Social Psychology* 4 (1966): 137–46; S. S. Kegeles, "Why People Seek Dental Care: A Test of a Conceptual Formulation," *Journal of Health and Human Behavior* 4 (Fall 1963): 166–73; J. P. Kirscht, "The Health Belief Model and Illness Behavior," *Health Education Monographs* 2 (1974): 387–408; M. Becker et al., "The Health Belief Model and Prediction of Dietary Compliance: A Field Experiment," *Journal of Health and Social Behavior* 18 (1977): 348–66.

7. M. Lalonde, *A New Perspective on the Health of Canadians* (Ottawa, Canada: Ministry of National Health and Welfare, 1974), p. 8.

8. L. Kohlberg, "Cognitive-Developmental Approach to Moral Education," *Humanist* 32, no. 6 (November-December 1972): 13–16; Carl A. Elder, *Making Value Judgements: Decisions of Today* (Chicago: Merrill, 1972); S. Simon, L. Howe, and H. Kirschenbaum, *Values Clarification: A Handbook of Practical Strategies for Teachers and Students* (New York: Hart, 1972); J. Osman, "The Use of Selected Value Clarifying Strategies in Health Education," *Journal of School Health* 54 (January 1974): 21–25.

9. R. Mucchielli, *Introduction to Structural Psychology* (New York: Funk & Wagnalls, 1970), p. 30.

10. Kirscht, "The Health Belief Model."

11. G. E. Osgood, G. J. Suci, and P. H. Tannenbaum, *The Measurement of Meaning* (Urbana: University of Illinois Press, 1961).

12. K. Sehnert and H. Eisenberg, *How to Be Your Own Doctor Sometimes* (New York: Grosset & Dunlap, 1975); D. Sobel and F. Hornbacher, *An Everyday Guide to Your Health* (New York: Grossman, 1973); G. S. Parcel, "Skills Approach to Health Education: A Framework for Integrating Cognitive and Affective Learning," *Journal of School Health* 66 (1976): 403–6; G. James, "The Effects of a Health Activation Program on Junior High School Students in Utah," *Health Education Monographs* 5 (Winter 1977): 380–81 (abstract).

13. N. Milio, "A Framework for Prevention: Changing Health-Damaging to Health-Generating Life Patterns," *American Journal of Public Health* 66 (May 1976), p. 436.

14. R. Jessor, "Predicting Time of Onset of Marijuana Use: A Developmental Study of High School Youth," in *Predicting Adolescent Drug Abuse: A Review of Issues, Methods and Correlates,* ed. D. J. Lettieri (National Institute of Drug Abuse, 1975).

15. D. Kandel, "Some Comments on the Relationship of Selected Criterion Variables to Adolescent Drug Use," ibid.

16. D. Mechanic, "The Influence of Mothers on Their Children's Health Attitudes and Behavior," *Pediatrics* 33 (March 1964): 444–53.

17. M. W. Kreuter, and L. W. Green, "Evaluation of School Health Education: Identifying Purpose, Keeping Perspective," *Journal of School Health* 48 (April 1978): 228–35.

18. W. A. Flexner, C. P. McLaughlin, and J. E. Littlefield, "Discovering What the Health Consumer Really Wants," *Health Care Management Reviews* 2 (Fall 1977): 43–49; L. W. Green, D. M. Levine, and S. G. Deeds, "Clinical Trials of Health Education for Hypertensive Outpatients: Design and Baseline Data," *Preventive Medicine* 4 (1975): 417–25.

19. A. L. Delbecq, A. H. Van de Ven, and D. A. Gustafson, *Group Techniques for Program Planning* (Glenview, Ill.: Scott, Foresman, 1975).

20. L. W. Green, "Should Health Education Abandon Attitude Change Strategies? Perspectives from Recent Research," *Health Education Monographs* 1, no. 30 (1970): 25–48; R. H. Aichlmayr, "Cultural Understanding: A Key to Acceptance," *Nursing Outlook* 17 (July 1969): 20–23; H. R. Robertson, "Removing Barriers to Health Care," ibid. (September 1969): 43–46.

21. L. W. Green and C. Kansler, *The Scientific and Professional Literature on Patient Education* (Detroit: Gale Information Service, 1979).

22. L. G. Reeder, L. Ramacher, and S. Gorednik, *The Handbook of Scales and Indices* (Santa Monica, Calif.: Goodyear, 1976).

23. L. A. Aday and R. Eichhorn, *The Utilization of Health Services: Indices and Correlates,* DHEW pub. no. (HRA) 73-3003, National Center for Health Services Research (1973).

24. M. Rokeach, *Beliefs, Attitudes and Values* (San Francisco: Jossey-Bass, 1970).

25. L. W. Green, "Diffusion and Adoption of Innovations Related to Cardiovascular Risk Behavior in the Public," in *Applying Behavioral Science to Cardiovascular Risk,* A. J. Enelow and J. B. Henderson, eds. (New York: American Heart Association, 1975); E. M. Rogers and F. F. Shoemaker, *Communication of Innovations: A Cross-Cultural Approach,* 2d ed. (New York: Free Press, 1971); E. M. Rogers, *Communication Strategies for Family Planning* (New York: Free Press, 1973).

CHAPTER 6

1. M. A. C. Young, *Review of Research and Studies Related to Health Education (1961–1966): Communication Methods and Materials, Health Education Monographs* 25 (1968):1–70; idem, *Review of Research and Studies Related to Health Education (1961–1966): Patient Education,* ibid. 26 (1968):1–64; idem, *Review of Research and*

Studies Related to Health Education Practice (1961–1966): School Health Education, ibid. 28 (1969): 1–97; C. H. Veenker, ed., *Synthesis of Research in Selected Areas of Health Instruction,* (Washington, D.C.: National Education Association, 1963).

2. J. M. Stephens, *The Process of Schooling: A Psychological Examination* (New York: Holt, 1967).

3. C. V. Good, ed., *Foundations in Education: Dictionary of Education* (New York: McGraw-Hill, 1959).

4. Young, "Review of Research: School Health Education"; Stephens, *The Process of Schooling;* J. E. Cauffman, "Effectiveness of Selected Approaches for the Teaching of Health Education," in *Synthesis of Research in Selected Areas of Health Instruction,* ed. C. H. Veenker (Washington, D.C.: National Education Association, 1963); P. L. Campeau, "Selective Review of the Results of Research on the Use of Audiovisual Media to Teach Adults," *Audio-Visual Communications Review* 22 (Spring 1974): 5–40.

5. Cauffman, "Effectiveness of Selected Approaches."

6. M. J. Gaines, "An Evaluation of Three Methods of Teaching Freshmen Health Education," *Journal of the American College Health Association* 13 (February 1965): 347–55.

7. L. W. Green, "Determining the Impact and Effectiveness of Health Education As It Relates to Federal Policy," *Health Education Monographs* 6, supplement no. 1 (1978): 28–66.

8. Idem, "Evaluation and Measurement: Some Dilemmas for Health Education," *American Journal of Public Health* 67 (February 1977): 155–61.

9. American Hospital Association, *Hospital Inpatient Education: Survey Findings and Analysis, 1975* (Atlanta: Bureau of Health Education, Center for Disease Control, 1977).

10. G. S. Wilkinson et al., "Measuring Response to a Cancer Information Telephone Facility: Can-Dial," *American Journal of Public Health* 66 (April 1976): 367–71; M. H. Bartlett, A. Johnston, and T. C. Mayer, "Dial Access Library—Patient Information Service," *New England Journal of Medicine* 288 (May 1973): 994–98.

11. H. Mendelsohn, "Mass Communications and Cancer Control," in *Cancer: The Behavioral Dimensions,* eds. J. W. Cullen et al. (New York: Raven, 1976).

12. W. Griffiths and A. L. Knutson, "The Role of Mass Media in Public Health," *American Journal of Public Health* 50 (April 1960): 515–23.

14. Surgeon General's Scientific Advisory Committee on Television and Social Behavior, *Television and Growing Up: The Impact of Televised Violence* (Public Health Service, 1972).

13. Green, "Determining Impact and Effectivenss of Health Education"; Griffiths and Knutson, "Mass Media in Public Health"; E. M. Rogers and F. F. Shoemaker, *Communication of Innovations: A Cross-Cultural Approach,* 2d ed. (New York: Free Press, 1971), pp. 346–85; E. M. Rogers, *Communication Strategies for Family Planning* (New York: Free Press, 1973); L. W. Green, "Diffusion and Adoption of Innovations Related to Cardiovascular Risk Behavior in the Public," in *Applying Behavioral Science to Cardiovascular Risk,* eds. A. Enelow and J. B. Henderson (New York: American Heart Association, 1975).

15. J. F. Engel, H. G. Wales, and M. R. Warshaw, *Promotional Strategy* (Homewood, Ill.: Irwin, 1975), pp. 223–70.

16. R. Betz, *A Taxonomy of Communication Media* (Englewood Cliffs, N.J.: Educational Technology, 1971).

17. A. C. McTaggart, "The Readability of Health Textbooks," in *Synthesis of Research in Selected Areas of Health Instruction,* ed. C. H. Veenker (Washington, D.C.: National Education Association, 1963).

18. R. R. Lanese and R. S. Thrush, "Measuring Readability of Health Education Literature," *Journal of American Dietetic Association* 42 (March 1963): 214–17; L. W. Green and R. R. Faden, "Patient-Package Inserts: Potential Impact on Patients," *Drug Information Journal* 2 (January 1977): 64s–70s (supplement); L. W. Green, "Educational Strategies to Improve Compliance with Preventive and Therapeutic Regimens: The Recent Evidence," in *Compliance in Health Care,* eds. R. B. Haynes, D. Sackett, and W. Taylor (Baltimore: Johns Hopkins University Press, 1979); F. Pyrczak and D. H. Roth, "The Readability of Directions on Nonprescription Drugs," *Journal of American Pharmacology Association* 16 (1976): 242–43, 267.

19. Cauffman, "Effectiveness of Selected Approaches."

20. Griffiths and Knutson, "Mass Media in Public Health."

21. P. L. Campeau, "Use of Audiovisual Media to Teach Adults."

22. H. I. Von Haden and J. M. King, *Educational Innovators' Guide* (Worthington, Ohio: James, 1974).

23. B. F. Skinner, "Teaching Machines," *Science* 128 (1958): 969–77.

24. A. G. Oettinger, *Run, Computer, Run! The Mythology of Educational Innovation* (Cambridge: Harvard University Press, 1969).

25. R. C. Butman, "CAI—There Is a Way to Make It Pay (But Not in Conventional Schooling)," *Educational Technology* 13 (December 1973): 5–9.

26. L. J. Van Cura et al., "Venereal Disease: Interviewing and Teaching by Computer," *American Journal of Public Health* 65 (1975): 1159–64; W. V. Slack et al., "Dietary Interviewing by Computer: An Experimental Approach to Counseling," *Journal of American Dietetic Association* 69 (1976): 514–17; L. A. Fisher et al., "Collection of a Clean Voided Urine Specimen: A Comparison Among Spoken, Written, and Computer-based Instructions," *American Journal of Public Health* 67 (July 1977): 640–44; D. Meadows, "Patients Learn About Diabetes from Teaching Machines," *Hospitals: JAHA* 39 (December 1965): 77–82.

27. M. E. Feldman, "Learning by Programmed and Test Format at Three Levels of Difficulty," *Journal of Educational Psychology* 56 (1965): 133–39; S. G. Owen et al., "Programmed Learning in Medical Education," *Postgraduate Medical Journal* 41 (1965): 201.

28. W. Schramm, "Learning from Instructional Television," *Review of Educational Research* 32 (1962): 156–57.

29. E. D. Schulz, "Television Brings Drama to Clinic Patients," *American Journal of Nursing* 62 (1962): 98–99.

30. Green, "Determining Impact and Effectiveness of Health Education."

31. Von Haden and King, *Educational Innovators' Guide.*

32. H. S. Barrows, "Simulated Patients (Programmed Patients)," in *The Development and Use of a New Technique in Medical Education* (Springfield, Ill.: Charles C Thomas, 1971).

33. D. A. Sleet and R. Stadsklev, "Annotated Bibliography of Simulations and Games in Health Education," *Health Education Monographs* 5, supplement no. 1 (1977).

34. J. S. Bruner, *Toward a Theory of Instruction* (Cambridge: Harvard University Press, 1966).

35. Cauffman, "Effectiveness of Selected Approaches."

36. R. Kaplan, "Teaching Problem-Solving with Television to College Freshmen in Health Education" (Ph.D. thesis, Ohio State University, 1962).

37. D. L. Roter, "Patient Participation in the Patient-Provider Interaction: The Effects of Patient Question-Asking on the Quality of Interaction, Satisfaction and Compliance," *Health Education Monographs* 5 (Winter 1977): 281–315.

38. K. Lewin, "Studies in Group Decision," in *Group Dynamics, Research and Theory,* eds. D. Cartwright and A. Zander (Evanston, Ill.: Row, Peterson, 1953).

39. B. Lubin and W. B. Eddy, "The Laboratory Training Model: Rationale, Method, and Some Thoughts for the Future," in *Sensitivity Training and the Laboratory Approach: Readings About Concepts and Applications,* eds. R. T. Golembiewski and A. Blumberg (Itasca, Ill.: Peacock, 1973).

40. B. W. Bond, *Group Discussion-Decision: An Appraisal of Its Use in Health Education* (Minneapolis: Minnesota Department of Health, 1956), pp. 1–109; idem, "A Study in Health Education Methods," *International Journal of Health Education* 1 (1958): 41–46.

41. V. L. Wang, "Application of Social Science Theories to Family Planning: Health Education in the People's Republic of China," *American Journal of Public Health* 66 (May 1976): 440–45.

42. Cauffman, "Effectiveness of Selected Approaches."

43. M. Radke and E. K. Caso, "Lecture and Discussion-Decision As Methods of Influencing Food Habits," *Journal of American Dietetic Association* 24 (January 1948): 23–31.

44. A. Bandura, "Social-learning Theory of Identificatory Processes," in *Handbook of Socialization Theory and Research,* ed. D. A. Goslin (Chicago: Rand McNally, 1969).

45. B. J. Zimmerman and T. L. Rosenthal, "Observational Learning of 'Rules' Governed Behavior by Children," *Psychological Bulletin* 81 (1974): 29–42.

46. A. Bandura, ed., *Psychological Modeling* (Chicago: Atherton, 1971).

47. J. L. Freedman, J. M. Carlsmith, and D. Q. Sears, *Social Psychology* (Englewood Cliffs, N.J.: Prentice-Hall, 1970), p. 239.

48. Surgeon General's Committee on Television and Behavior, *Impact of Televised Violence.*

49. L. W. Green, "Should Health Education Abandon Attitude Change Strategies? Perspectives from Recent Research," *Health Education Monographs* 1, no. 30, (1970): 25–48.

50. M. J. Mahoney, *Cognition and Behavior Modification* (Cambridge, Mass.: Ballinger, 1974); D. L. Watson and R. G. Tharp, *Self-Directed Behavior—Self-Modification for Personal Adjustment* (Monterey, Calif.: Brooks/Cole, 1977).

51. R. C. Katz and S. Zlutnick, eds., *Behavior Therapy and Health Care Principles and Applications* (New York: Pergamon, 1975).

52. J. P. Foreyt, ed., *Behavioral Treatment of Obesity* (Oxford: Pergamon, 1977).
53. F. Bass, "Behavior Modification: A Review of Basic Concepts and Recent Research," in *Health Promotion and Consumer Health Education: Preventive Medicine, USA,* Fogarty International Center and the American College of Preventive Medicine (New York: Prodist, 1976).
54. Mahoney, *Cognition and Behavior Modification.*
55. J. Rothman, "Three Models of Community Organization Practice," in *Strategies of Community Organization: A Book of Readings,* eds. F. M. Cox et al. (Itasca, Ill.: Peacock, 1970).
56. H. C. Johnston, "Health Education in the Extension Service: A Historical Perspective," *Health Education Monographs* 3 (Spring 1975): 13–25.
57. R. H. Grant, "Family and Self-Help Education in Isolated Rural Communities," ibid. 5 (Summer 1977): 143–60.
58. V. E. Hamilton, "Community Resource Development: Health Education Programs in North Carolina," in *Proceedings: Extension Seminar on Health Education and Rural Health Care Research Forum,* ed. B. L. Bible (Chicago: American Medical Association, 1976).
59. N. M. Clark and A. Wolderfael, "Community Development Through Integration of Services and Education," *International Journal of Health Education* 20 (1977): 189–99.
60. A. V. Dominguez, "Stimulating Community Involvement Through Mass Organizations in Cuba: The Women's Role," *International Journal of Health Education* 20 (1977): 57–60; T. Drummond, *Using the Method of Paulo Freire in Nutrition Education: An Experimental Plan for Community Action in Northeast Brazil,* Cornell International Nutrition Monograph Series no. 3 (Ithaca, N.Y.: Cornell University Press, 1975); B. Tomic et al., "Ivanjica: A Community Conquers Health," *International Journal of Health Education* 20 (1977): 1–16, supplement; H. A. K. Kanaaneh et al., "The Eradication of a Large Scabies Outbreak Using Community-wide Health Education," *American Journal of Public Health* 66 (June 1976): 564–67; L. P. Medis and P. A. Fernando, "Health Education in Emergency Situations: A Cholera Outbreak in Sri Lanka," *International Journal of Health Education* 20 (1977): 200–204.
61. L. W. Green et al., "Research and Demonstration Issues in Self-care: Measuring the Decline of Medicocentrism," *Health Education Monographs* 5 (Summer 1977): 161–89; L. S. Levin et al., *Self-care: Lay Initiatives in Health* (New York: Prodist, 1976).
62. Rothman, "Community Organization Practice."
63. Ibid.
64. W. L. French and C. H. Bell, *Organizational Development: Behavioral Science Interventions for Organization Improvement* (Englewood Cliffs, N.J.: Prentice-Hall, 1973).
65. W. W. Burke and H. A. Hornstein, eds., *The Social Technology of Organizational Development* (Fairfax, Va.: National Learning Resources, 1972).
66. P. R. Mico and H. S. Ross, *Health Education and Behavioral Science* (Oakland: Third Party, 1975).
67. Society for Public Health Education, *Training, Health Education Monographs* 3 (Fall 1975); M. C. Thorne, ed., *Consultation,* ibid. 4 (Winter 1975).

68. J. M. Metsch et al., "The Impact of Training on Consumer Participation in the Delivery of Health Services," ibid. (Fall 1975): 251–61.
69. N. M. Clark and M. Pinkett-Heller, "Developing HSA Leadership: An Innovation in Board Education," *American Journal of Health Planning* 2 (July 1977): 9–13.
70. W. Carlton, "The Health Team Training Model: A Teaching-Learning Approach in Community Health," *Health Education Monographs* 5 (Spring 1977): 62–74.
71. P. M. Lazes et al., "Improving Patient Care Through Participation: The Newark Experiment in Staff and Patient Involvement," *International Journal of Health Education* 20 (1977): 61–68.

CHAPTER 7

1. Mary F. Arnold, *Health Program Implementation Through PERT—Administrative and Educational Uses,* Continuing Education monograph no. 6 (San Francisco: American Public Health Association, 1966).
2. Gerald Zaltman and Robert Duncan, *Strategies for Planned Change* (New York: Wiley, 1977); Warren G. Bennis, *Changing Organization* (New York: McGraw-Hill, 1966); Richard Beckhard, *Organization Development: Strategies and Models* (Reading, Mass.: Addison-Wesley, 1966); R. G. Havelock and M. G. Havelock, *Training for Change Agents* (Ann Arbor: Institute for Social Research, University of Michigan Press, 1973); J. Rothman, J. Erlich, and J. G. Teresa, *Promoting Innovation and Change in Organizations and Communities* (New York: Wiley, 1976); I. Rubin, M. Plovnik, and R. Fry, "Initiating Planned Changes in Health Care Systems," *Journal of Applied Behavioral Science* 10 (1974): 107–124; Warren G. Bennis et al., *The Planning of Change,* 3d ed. (New York: Holt, 1976).
3. L. W. Green et al., *The Dacca Family Planning Experiment: A Comparative Evaluation of Programs Directed at Males and at Females,* Pacific Health Education Reports, no. 3 (Berkeley: University of California Press, 1972); L. W. Green, D. M. Levine, and S. G. Deeds, "Clinical Trials of Health Education for Hypertensive Outpatients: Design and Baseline Data." *Preventive Medicine* 4 (1975): 417–25.
4. Harold Wise et al., *Making Health Teams Work* (New York: Ballinger, 1974); Alberta Parker, *The Team Approach to Primary Care,* Neighborhood Health Center Seminar Program Monograph Series no. 3 (Berkeley: University of California, January 1972); Richard Beckhard, "Organizational Issues in the Team Delivery of Comprehensive Health Care," *Milbank Memorial Fund Quarterly* 1, no. 3, pt. 1 (July 1972): 287–316.
5. Kay B. Partridge, "Planning a Health Education Program. The Critical Role of Situational Analysis," *Proceedings. Patient Education Workshop,* Health Education Center, Oct. 29, 1975 (Baltimore: Health Education Center, Maryland State Department of Health and Mental Hygiene, 1976), pp. 9–22.
6. *Putting Knowledge to Use: A Distillation of the Literature Regarding Knowledge Transfer and Change* (Los Angeles, Calif.: Human Interaction Research Institute, 1976), pp. 5–8.
7. Ibid.

8. L. W. Green et al., *Guidelines for Health Education in Maternal and Child Health, International Journal of Health Education* 21 (supplement) no. 3 (July–September 1978): 1–33.

CHAPTER 8

1. John B. Atwater, "Adapting the Venereal Disease Clinic to Today's Problem," *American Journal of Public Health* 64 (May 1974): 433–37.
2. Jerald Bailey, "An Evaluative Look at a Family Planning Radio Campaign in Latin America," *Studies in Family Planning* 4 (October 1973): 275–78; Laura E. Edwards et al., "An Experimental Comprehensive High School Clinic," *American Journal of Public Health* 67 (August 1977): 765–66; L. W. Green et al., "Research and Demonstration Issues in Self-care: Measuring the Decline of Medicocentrism," *Health Education Monographs* 5 (Summer 1977): 161–85; E. Hyock Kwon, "Use of the Agent System in Seoul," *Studies in Family Planning* 2 (November 1971): 237–340; S. S. Lieberman, "The Isfahan Communication Project," ibid. 4 (April 1973): 87–91; Lillian D. Long, "The Evaluation of Continuing Education Efforts," *American Journal of Public Health* 59 (June 1969): 967–73; Noralou P. Roos, "Evaluating Health Programs: Where Do We Find the Data?" *Journal of Community Health* 1 (Fall 1975): 39–51; Charlotte V. Spiegel and Francis C. Lindaman, "Children Can't Fly: A Program to Prevent Childhood Morbidity and Mortality from Window Falls," *American Journal of Public Health* 67 (December 1977): 143–47; Kenneth E. Warner, "The Effects of the Anti-Smoking Campaign on Cigarette Consumption," ibid. (July 1977): 645–50.
3. J. G. Brennan et al., "Continuing Education in Alcoholism: Attitude Change As a Measure of Seminar Effectiveness," *Maryland State Medical Journal* 23 (1974): 63–67; Robert H. Conn and Dudley Anderson, "D.C. Mounts Unfunded Program of Screening for Lead Poisoning," *HSMHA Health Report* 86 (May 1971): 409–13; Daniel Rosenblatt and Levon Kabasakalian, "Evaluation of Venereal Disease Information Campaign for Adolescents," *American Journal of Public Health* 56 (July 1966): 1104–14; John Williamson et al., "Health Accounting: An Outcome-based System of Quality Assurance—Illustrative Applications to Hypertension," *Bulletin of the New York Academy of Medicine* 51 (1975): 727–38.
4. L. W. Green and K. J. Krotki, "Class and Parity Biases in Family Planning Programs: The Case of Karachi," *Eugenics Quarterly (Social Biology)* 15 (December 1968): 235–51; J. S. Neill and J. O. Bond, *Hillsborough County Oral Polio Vaccine Program,* Florida State Board of Health monograph no. 6 (Jacksonville: Florida State Board of Health, 1964); V. L. Wang, Paul Ephross, and L. W. Green, "The Point of Diminishing Returns in Nutrition Education Through Home Visits by Aides: An Evaluation of EFNEP," *Health Education Monographs* 3 (Spring 1975): 70–88; G. H. Ward, "Changing Trends in Control of Hypertension," *Public Health Reports* 93 (January–February 1978): 31–34.
5. John W. Farquhar et al., "Community Education for Cardiovascular Health," *Lancet* 1, no. 8023 (June 4, 1977): 1192–95.
6. L. W. Green et al., *The Dacca Family Planning Experiment: A Comparative Evaluation of Programs Directed at Males and at Females,* Pacific Health Education Reports,

no. 3 (Berkeley: University of California Press, 1972); N. Maccoby et al., "Reducing the Risk of Cardiovascular Disease: Effects of a Community-based Campaign on Knowledge and Behavior," *Journal of Community Health* 3 (Winter 1977): 100–114; Beryl J. Roberts et al., "An Experimental Study of Two Approaches to Communication," *American Journal of Public Health* 53 (September 1963): 1361–81; Sidney Stahl et al., "Motivational Interventions in Community Hypertension Screening," ibid. 67 (April 1977): 345–52; Sheldon S. Steinberg and Eugene D. Fitzpatrick, "The Paducah Health Education Survey, 1958," ibid. 51 (May 1961): 732–45; G. S. Wilkinson et al., "Measuring Response to a Cancer Information Telephone Facility: Can-Dial," ibid. 66 (April 1976): 367–71.

7. Robert A. Dershewitz and John W. Williamson, "Preventing of Childhood Household Injuries: A Controlled Clinical Trial," *American Journal of Public Health* 67 (December 1977): 1148–53; James F. Phillips et al., "An Experiment with Payment, Quota, and Clinic Affiliation Schemes for Lay Motivators in the Philippines," *Studies in Family Planning* 6 (September 1975): 326–34; Emerson Robinson, "A Comparative Evaluation of the Scrub and Brush Methods of Toothbrushing with Flossing As an Adjunct (in Fifth- and Sixth-Graders)," *American Journal of Public Health* 66 (November 1976): 1078–81; D. L. Roter, "Patient Participation in the Patient-Provider Interaction: The Effects of Patient Question-Asking on the Quality of Interaction, Satisfaction and Compliance," *Health Education Monographs* 5 (Winter 1977): 281–315; J. Sayegh and L. W. Green, "Family Planning Education: Program Design, Training Component and Cost-Effectiveness of a Postpartum Program in Beirut," *International Journal of Health Education* 19 (January–March 1976): 1–20 (supplement); P. B. Smith et al., "The Medical Impact of an Antepartum Program for Pregnant Adolescents: A Statistical Analysis," *American Journal of Public Health* 78 (February 1978): 169–72.

8. Jerald Bailey and Maria Cristinade Zambrano, "Contraceptive Pamphlets in Colombian Drugstores," *Studies in Family Planning* 5 (June 1974): 178–82; Irene Dalzell, "Evaluation of a Prenatal Teaching Program," *Nursing Research* 14 (Spring 1965): 160–63; T. W. Elwood, E. Ericson, and S. Lieberman, "Comparative Educational Approaches to Screening for Colorectal Cancer," *American Journal of Public Health* 68 (February 1978): 135–38; A. A. Fisher et al., "Training Teachers in Population Education Institutes in Baltimore," *Journal of School Health* 46 (September 1976): 357–60; L. W. Green, D. M. Levine, and S. G. Deeds, "Clinical Trials of Health Education for Hypertensive Outpatients: Design and Baseline Data," *Preventive Medicine* 4 (1975): 417–25; M. J. Kupst et al., "Evaluation of Methods to Improve Communication in the Physician-Patient Relationship," *American Journal of Orthopsychiatry* 45 (April 1975): 420–29; Ruanne Peters et al., "Daily Relaxation Response Breaks in a Working Population: II. Effects on Blood Pressure," *American Journal of Public Health* 67 (October 1977): 954–59.

9. L. W. Green, "Evaluation and Measurement: Some Dilemmas for Health Education," *American Journal of Public Health* 67 (February 1977): 155–61.

10. D. A. Bertram and P. A. Brooks-Bertram, "The Evaluation of Continuing Medical Education: A Literature Review," *Health Education Monographs* 5 (Winter 1977): 330–62; I. Figà-Talamanca, "Problems in the Evaluation of Training of Health Personnel," ibid. 3 (Fall 1975): 232–50; M. W. Kreuter and L. W. Green, "Evaluation of School Health Education: Identifying Purpose,

Keeping Perspective," *Journal of School Health* 48 (April 1978): 228–35; Guy W. Steuart, "Planning and Evaluation in Health Education," *International Journal of Health Education* 12 (1969): 65–76.

CHAPTER 9

1. V. Wang, P. Ephross, and L. W. Green, "The Point of Diminishing Returns in Nutrition Education Through Home Visits by Aides: An Evaluation of EFNEP," *Health Education Monographs* 3 (Spring 1975): 70–88; S. Rymer, "A Community Health Representative Program," *Health Education* 7 (November–December 1976): 17–19.
2. A. S. Castile and S. Jerrick, *School Health in America, A Survey of School Health Programs* (Kent, Ohio: American School Health Association, 1976).
3. E. M. Sliepcevich, *School Health Education Study: A Summary Report* (Washington, D.C.: School Health Education Study, 1964).
4. R. D. Russell, *Health Education* (Washington, D.C.: National Education Association, 1975).
5. *School Health Curriculum Project*, DHEW pub. no. (CDC) 78-8359 (December 1977).
6. Ibid.
7. F. Kunstel, "Assessing Community Needs: Implications for Curriculum and Staff Development in Health Education," *Journal of School Health* 48 (April 1978): 220–24.
8. G. W. Comstock and J. A. Tonascia, "Education and Mortality in Washington County, Maryland," *Journal of Health and Social Behavior* 18 (March 1977): 54–61.
9. G. Botvin, A. Eng, and C. L. Williams, "Preventing the Onset of Smoking Through Life Skills Training" (Paper prepared for the American Health Foundation, 1979).
10. H. Benson, "Systemic Hypertension and the Relaxation Response," *New England Journal of Medicine* 296 (May 19, 1977): 1152–56.
11. R. C. Knott, "Health Activities Project—A Different Approach" (Paper presented at the annual meeting of the American School Health Association, Atlanta, October 1977).
12. C. E. Lewis and M. A. Lewis, quoted in *Health Promotion and Consumer Health Education: Preventive Medicine, USA. A Task Force Report by NIH and American College of Preventive Medicine,* Fogarty International Center and the American College of Preventive Medicine (New York: Prodist, 1976).
13. G. S. Parcel, "Skills Approach to Health Education: A Framework for Integrating Cognitive and Affective Learning," *Journal of School Health* 66 (1976): 403–6.
14. P. Heit, "The Berkeley Model," *Health Education* 8 (January–February 1977): 2–3; G. James, "The Effects of a Health Activation Program on Junior High School Students in Utah," *Health Education Monographs* 5 (Winter 1977): 380–81 (abstract).
15. E. M. Rogers and F. F. Shoemaker, *Communication of Innovations: A Cross-Cultural Approach* (New York: Free Press, 1971).

16. R. I. Evans et al., "Deterring the Onset of Smoking in Children: Knowledge of Immediate Physiological Effects and Coping with Peer Pressure, Media Pressure and Parent Modeling," *Journal of Applied Social Psychology* 8, no. 2 (1978): 126–35.

17. A. McAlister, "Systematic Peer Leadership to Discourage Onset of Tobacco Dependency" (Paper presented at the annual meeting of the American Psychological Association, Toronto, August 1978).

CHAPTER 10

1. The Nursing Development Conference Group, *Concept Formalization in Nursing: Process and Product* (Boston: Little, Brown, 1973).

2. R. Schlotfeldt, "This I Believe . . . Nursing Is Health Care," *Nursing Outlook* 30 (April 1972): 245.

3. American Nurses' Association, *Facts About Nursing '74–'75* (Kansas City, Mo.: American Nurses' Association, 1976), p. 3.

4. B. K. Redman, *The Process of Patient Teaching in Nursing,* 3d ed. (St. Louis: Mosby, 1976); V. Henderson and G. Nite, *Principles and Practice of Nursing* (New York: Macmillan, 1978).

5. A. Ackerman et al., "Survey of Health Education in Nursing Practice," mimeographed (Baltimore, Md.: Division of Health Education, School of Hygiene and Public Health, Johns Hopkins University, 1978).

6. S. E. Archer and R. Fleshman, *Community Health Nursing* (Belmont, Calif.: Wadsworth, 1975); R. B. Freeman, *Community Health Nursing Practice* (Philadelphia: Saunders, 1970); C. W. Tinkham and E. F. Voorhies, *Community Health Nursing Evolution and Process* (New York: Appleton-Century-Crofts, 1972); A. M. Reinhardt and M. D. Quinn, eds., *Current Practices in Family-Centered Community Nursing,* vol. 1 (St. Louis: Mosby, 1977).

7. A. M. Reinhardt and E. D. Chatlin, "Assessment of Health Needs in a Community: The Basis for Program Planning," in *Current Practices in Family-Centered Community Nursing,* eds. A. M. Reinhardt and M. D. Quinn (St. Louis: Mosby, 1977), pp. 138–90.

8. Henderson and Nite, *Principles of Nursing;* F. L. Bower, *The Process of Planning Nursing Care* (St. Louis: Mosby, 1972); L. W. Green et al., "Research and Demonstration Issues in Self-care: Measuring the Decline of Medicocentrism," *Health Education Monographs* 5 (Summer 1977): 161–89.

9. Bower, *Planning Nursing Care.*

10. Ackerman et al., *Survey of Health Education;* H. Yura and M. B. Walsh, *The Nursing Process,* 2d ed. (New York: Appleton-Century-Crofts, 1973).

11. Reinhardt and Quinn, *Family-Centered Nursing;* C. Williams, "Community Health Nursing—What Is It?," *Nursing Outlook* 25 (April 1977): 250–54; V. Ruth and K. B. Partridge, "Community Health Nursing: Differences in Perception of Education and Practice," ibid. 26 (October 1978): 622–28.

12. S. Jencks and L. W. Green, "Developing a Hospital-based Patient Education Program," *Quality Review Bulletin* 4 (October 1978): 8–11.

13. Henderson and Nite, *Principles of Nursing.*

APPENDIX B

1. "Health Education Strategies for Hypertension Control," National Heart, Lung, and Blood Institute grant no. 1R25HL17016, co-principle investigators L. W. Green and D. M. Levine, Johns Hopkins Health Services Research and Development Center, 1974.

2. J. Stamler et al., "Hypertension. The Problem and the Challenge," in *The Hypertension Handbook* (West Point, Pa.: Merck Sharp & Dohme, 1974), 3–29.

3. *Hypertension and Hypertensive Heart Disease in Adults, United States, 1960–62,* National Health Survey, National Center for Health Statistics, series 11, no. 13 (1966).

4. I. M. Moriyama, D. E. Kreuger, and J. Stamler, *Cardiovascular Diseases in the United States* (Cambridge, Mass.: Harvard University Press, 1971), p. 119.

5. *Social Security Disability Applicant Statistics, 1968,* DHEW pub. no. (SSA) 73-1911 Social Security Administration, Office of Research and Statistics (June 1972).

6. Stamler et al., "Hypertension," p. 27.

7. Veterans Administration Cooperative Study Group on Antihypertensive Agents: Effects of Treatment on Morbidity in Hypertension, "1. Results in Patients with Diastolic Blood Pressure Averaging 115 Through 129 mm Hg," *Journal of American Medical Association* 202 (1967):1028; idem, "II. Results in Patients with Diastolic Blood Pressures Averaging 90 Through 114 mm Hg," ibid. 213 (1970):1143; idem, "Influence of Age, Diastolic Pressure, and Prior Cardiovascular Disease: Further Analysis of Side Effects," *Circulation* 45 (1972): 991.

8. Stamler et al., "Hypertension."

9. Inter-Society Commission for Heart Disease Resources, Atherosclerosis Study Group and Epidemiology Study Group, "Primary Prevention of the Atherosclerotic Diseases," *Circulation* 42 (1970): A55; *The Health and Nutrition Examination Survey 1971* (preliminary data), DHEW pub. no. (NIH) 77-1216 National High Blood Pressure Education Program (1977); *Fourteen Communities Survey, February 1973–June 1974, Hypertension Detection and Follow-up Study,* National Heart, Lung, and Blood Institute, quoted in *The National High Blood Pressure Month Book, May 1977,* NHBPEP, DHEW pub. no. (NIH) 77-1216 (1977).

10. Inter-Society Commission for Heart Disease Resources, "Primary Prevention of Atherosclerotic Diseases"; idem, "Guidelines for the Detection, Diagnosis, and Management of Hypertensive Populations," *Circulation* 44 (1971): A263, rev. August 1972.

11. L. W. Green, F. M. Lewis, and D. M. Levine, "The Complementarity of Statistical Profiles, Clinical Judgement, and Behavioral Theory in the Diagnosis of Patient Educational Needs" (Paper presented at the Second Annual Needs Assessment Conference, Louisville, Ky., March 28, 1978).

12. T. S. Inui, "Effects of Post-Graduate Physician Education on the Management and Outcomes of Patients with Hypertension" (Sc.M. thesis, Johns Hopkins University School of Hygiene and Public Health, 1973).

13. L. W. Green, D. M. Levine, and S. G. Deeds, "Clinical Trials of Health Education for Hypertensive Outpatients: Design and Baseline Data," *Preventive Medicine* 4 (1975): 417–25.

14. Green, Lewis, and Levine, "Complementarity in the Diagnosis of Educational Needs"; Green, Levine, and Deeds, "Clinical Trials of Health Education for Hy-

pertensive Outpatients"; L. W. Green et al., "Development of Randomized Patient Education Experiments with Urban Poor Hypertensives," *Patient Counseling and Health Education* 1 (Winter/Spring 1979): 106–11.

15. Green, Levine, and Deeds, "Clinical Trials of Health Education for Hypertensive Outpatients."

16. Green et al., "Randomized Experiments with Urban Poor Hypertensives."

17. Ibid.

18. L. Gordis, M. Markowitz, and A. Lilienfeld, "The Inaccuracy of Using Interviews to Estimate Patient Reliability in Taking Medications at Home," *Medical Care* 7 (1969): 49–54; D. L. Sackett and R. B. Haynes, *Compliance with Therapeutic Regimens* (Baltimore: Johns Hopkins University Press, 1976).

19. Green et al., "Randomized Experiments with Urban Poor Hypertensives."

20. R. H. Brook, "A Study of the Methodologic Problems Associated with Assessment of Quality of Care" (Sc.D. diss., Johns Hopkins University School of Hygiene and Public Health, 1972).

21. Inui, "Effects of Physician Education on Patients with Hypertension."

22. Ibid.

23. Green et al., "Randomized Experiments with Urban Poor Hypertensives."

24. S. G. Deeds et al., "Incorporating a Hospital Systems Analysis into Patient Education Research," Johns Hopkins Health Services Research and Development Center, 1978.

25. Green, Levine, and Deeds, "Clinical Trials of Health Education for Hypertensive Outpatients"; Green et al., Randomized Experiments with Urban Poor Hypertensives."

26. Green, Levine, and Deeds, Clinical Trials of Health Education for Hypertensive Outpatients; D. M. Levine et al., "Health Education for Hypertensive Patients," *Journal of American Medical Association* 241 (April 20, 1979): 1700–03.

27. Green et al., "Randomized Experiments with Urban Poor Hypertensives."

28. Ibid.

29. Ibid.; Levine et al., "Health Education for Hypertensive Patients."

30. Green, Lewis, and Levine, "Complementarity in the Diagnosis of Educational Needs."

31. B. G. Glaser and A. L. Strauss, *Grounded Theory* (Chicago: Aldine, 1965); P. D. Mullen, "Cutting Back: An Overview," *Health Education Monographs,* in press.

32. M. H. Becker and L. W. Green, "A Family Approach to Compliance with Medical Regimens: A Selective Review of the Literature," *International Journal of Health Education* 18, no. 3 (July–September 1975): 173–82.

33. M. F. Fass, L. W. Green, and D. M. Levine, "Design of an Experimental Intervention to Increase Family Reinforcement in the Home for Patient Compliance" (Paper presented at the 103d Annual Meeting of the American Public Health Association, Chicago, November 1975).

34. B. S. Wallston et al., "Development and Validation of the Health Locus of Control (HLC) Scale," *Journal of Consulting and Clinical Psychology* 44 (August 1976): 580–85. See also K. A. Wallston and B. S. Wallston, eds., *Locus of Control and Health: A Review of the Literature, Health Education Monographs* 6, no. 2 (Spring 1978): 107–17.

35. Levine et al., "Health Education for Hypertensive Patients"; Fass, Green, and Levine, "Experimental Intervention to Increase Family Reinforcement"; A. J. Chwalow et al., "Exit Interviews As a First Stage in Patient Education to Improve Compliance with Hypertension Regimens" (Paper presented at a meeting of the American Public Health Association, Chicago, Ill., 1975); M. Bowler, "Internality Training and Compliance Behavior of Hypertensive Patients," (Ph.D. diss., Washington University, 1978).

36. Wallston et al., "Development and Validation of the Health Locus of Control (HLC) Scale."

37. Levine et al., "Health Education for Hypertensive Patients."

Bibliography

Abudejaja, A. H. "Some Determinants of Compliance with Treatment Following Blood Pressure Screening." Ph.D. dissertation, Johns Hopkins University School of Hygiene and Public Health, 1978.

Ackerman, A., and Kalmer, H. "Health Education and Baccalaureate Nursing Curriculum—Myth or Reality." Paper presented at the 105th Annual Meeting of the American Public Health Association, 1 November 1977, Washington, D.C.

Ackerman, A., et al. "Survey of Health Education in Nursing Practice." Mimeographed. Baltimore, Md.: Division of Health Education, School of Hygiene and Public Health Johns Hopkins University, 1978.

Aday, L. A., and Eichhorn, R. *The Utilization of Health Services: Indices and Correlates.* DHEW pub. no. (HRA) 73-3003. National Center for Health Services Research, 1973.

Aichlmayr, R. H. "Cultural Understanding: A Key to Acceptance." *Nursing Outlook* 17 (July 1969): 20–23.

American Hospital Association. *Hospital Inpatient Education: Survey Findings and Analysis, 1975.* Atlanta: Bureau of Health Education, Center for Disease Control, 1977.

277

American Nurses' Association. *Facts About Nursing '74–'75*. Kansas City, Mo.: American Nurses' Association, 1976.

Andersen, R. *A Behavioral Model of Families' Use of Health Services*. University of Chicago Center for Health Administration Studies Research Series, no. 25. Chicago: University of Chicago Press, 1968.

Anderson, C. I.; Morton, R; and Green, L. W. *Community Health*. 3rd ed. St. Louis: Mosby, 1978.

Archer, S. E., and Fleshman, R. *Community Health Nursing*. Belmont, Calif.: Wadsworth, 1975.

Arnold, Mary F. *Health Program Implementation Through PERT–Administrative and Educational Uses*. Continuing Education monograph no. 6. San Francisco: American Public Health Association, 1966.

Atwater, John B. "Adapting the Venereal Disease Clinic to Today's Problem." *American Journal of Public Health* 64 (May 1974): 433–37.

Bailey, Jerald. "An Evaluative Look at a Family Planning Radio Campaign in Latin America." *Studies in Family Planning* 4 (October 1973): 275–78.

Bailey, Jerald, and Zambrano, Maria Cristinade. "Contraceptive Pamphlets in Colombian Drugstores." *Studies in Family Planning* 5 (June 1974): 178–82.

Bandura, A. "Social-learning Theory of Identificatory Processes." In *Handbook of Socialization Theory and Research,* edited by D. A. Goslin. Chicago, Rand McNally, 1969.

Bandura, A., ed. *Psychological Modeling*. Chicago: Atherton, 1971.

Barrows, H. S. "Simulated Patients (Programmed Patients)." In *The Development and Use of a New Technique in Medical Education*. Springfield, Ill.: Charles C Thomas, 1971.

Bartlett, M. H.; Johnston, A; and Mayer, T. C. "Dial Access Library—Patient Information Service." *New England Journal of Medicine* 288 (May 1973): 994–98.

Baselines for Setting Health Goals and Standards. DHEW pub. no. (HRA) 77-640. Health Resources Administration, 1977.

Bass, F. "Behavior Modification: A Review of Basic Concepts and Recent Research." In *Health Promotion and Consumer Health Education: Preventive Medicine, USA,* Fogarty International Center and the American College of Preventive Medicine. New York: Prodist, 1976.

Becker, M., et al. "The Health Belief Model and Prediction of Dietary Compliance: A Field Experiment." *Journal of Health and Social Behavior* 18 (1977): 348–66.

Becker, M. H., and Green, L. W. "A Family Approach to Compliance with Medical Regimens: A Selective Review of the Literature." *International Journal of Health Education* 18, no. 3 (July–September 1975): 173–82.

Beckhard, Richard. *Organization Development: Strategies and Models*. Reading, Mass.: Addison-Wesley, 1966.

Beckhard, Richard. "Organizational Issues in the Team Delivery of Comprehensive Health Care." *Milbank Memorial Fund Quarterly* 1, no. 3, pt. 1 (July 1972): 287–316.

Bennett, B. I. "A Model for Teaching Health Education Skills to Primary Care Practitioners." *International Journal of Health Education* 20, no. 4 (1977): 232–39.

Bennis, Warren G. *Changing Organization.* New York: McGraw-Hill, 1966.

Bennis, Warren G., et al. *The Planning of Change,* 3d ed. New York: Holt 1976.

Benson, H. "Systemic Hypertension and the Relaxation Response." *New England Journal of Medicine* 296 (May 19, 1977): 1152–56.

Berry, R. E., Jr., and Boland, J. P. *The Economic Cost of Alcohol Abuse and Alcoholism.* Boston: Policy Analysis, 1974.

Bertram, D. A., and Brooks-Bertram, P. A. "The Evaluation of Continuing Medical Education: A Literature Review." *Health Education Monographs* 5 (Winter 1977): 330–62.

Betz, R. *A Taxonomy of Communication Media.* Englewood Cliffs, N.J.: Educational Technology, 1971.

Blockstein, W. L.; Bailey, A. R.; and Hansen, R. H. "Expanding the Role of a University in Consumer Health Education." *Health Education Monographs* 3 (Spring 1975): 62–69.

Bond, B. W. *Group Discussion-Decision: An Appraisal of Its Use in Health Education.* Minneapolis: Minnesota Department of Health, 1956.

Bond, B. W. "A Study in Health Education Methods. "*International Journal of Health Education* 1 (1958): 41–46.

Borhani, N. O. "Primary Prevention of Coronary Heart Disease: A Critique."*American Journal of Cardiology* 40 (August 1977): 251–59.

Botvin, G., Eng, A., and Williams, C. L. "Preventing the Onset of Smoking Through Life Skills Training." Paper prepared for the American Health Foundation, 1979.

Bowler, M. "Internality Training and Compliance Behavior of Hypertensive Patients," Ph.D. dissertation, Washington University, 1978.

Bowman, M. L. C. "Assessing College Student Attitudes Toward Environmental Issues." *Journal of Environmental Education* 6 (Winter 1974): 1–5.

Bradburn, N., and Capolvitz, D. *Reports on Happiness: A Pilot Study of Behavior Related to Mental Health.* New York: Aldine, 1965.

Brennan, J. G., et al. "Continuing Education in Alcoholism: Attitude Change As a Measure of Seminar Effectiveness." *Maryland State Medical Journal* 23 (1974): 63–67.

Brook, R. H. "A Study of the Methodologic Problems Associated with Assessment of Quality of Care." Sc.D. dissertation, Johns Hopkins University School of Hygiene and Public Health, 1972.

Bruess, C., and Gay, J. *Implementing Comprehensive School Health.* New York: Macmillan, 1978.

Bruner, J. S. *Toward a Theory of Instruction.* Cambridge: Harvard University Press, 1966.

Burke, W. W., and Hornstein, H. A., eds. *The Social Technology of Organizational Development.* Fairfax, Va.: National Learning Resources, 1972.

Butman, R. C. "CAI—There Is a Way to Make It Pay (But Not in Conventional Schooling)." *Educational Technology* 13 (December 1973): 5–9.

Campbell, A.; Converse, P. E.; and Rodgers, W. L. *The Quality of American Life: Perceptions, Evaluations and Satisfaction.* New York: Russell Sage, 1976.

Campeau, P. L. "Selective Review of the Results of Research on the Use of Audio-visual Media to Teach Adults." *Audiovisual Communications Review* 22 (Spring 1974): 5–40.

Carlton, W. "The Health Team Training Model: A Teaching-Learning Approach in Community Health." *Health Education Monographs* 5 (Spring 1977): 62–74.

Cartwright, D. "Some Principles of Mass Persuasion: Selected Findings from Research on the Sale of United States War Bonds." *Human Relations* 2 (1949): 253–69.

Castile, A. S., and Jerrick, S. *School Health in America, A Survey of School Health Programs.* Kent, Ohio: American School Health Association, 1976.

Cauffman, J. E. "Effectiveness of Selected Approaches for the Teaching of Health Education." In *Synthesis of Research in Selected Areas of Health Instruction,* edited by C. H. Veenker. Washington, D.C.: National Education Association, 1963.

Chun, K. T.; Cobb, S.; and French, J. R. P., Jr. *Measures for Psychological Assessment: A Guide to 3,000 Original Sources and Their Applications.* Ann Arbor: University of Michigan Institute for Social Research, 1975.

Chwalow, A. J. "Contact vs. Content: The Effect of the Multiplicity of Health Education Encounters on Compliance and Blood Pressure Control." Dr.P.H. dissertation, Johns Hopkins University School of Hygiene and Public Health, 1978.

Chwalow, A. J., et al. "Exit Interviews As a First Stage in Patient Education to Improve Compliance with Hypertension Regimens." Paper presented at a meeting of the American Public Health Association, 1975, Chicago, Ill.

Clark, N. M., and Pinkett-Heller, M. "Developing HSA Leadership: An Innovation in Board Education." *American Journal of Health Planning* 2 (July 1977): 9–13.

Clark, N. M., and Wolderfael, A. "Community Development Through Integration of Services and Education." *International Journal of Health Education* 20 (1977): 189–99.

Comstock, G. W., and Tonascia, J. A. "Education and Mortality in Washington County, Maryland." *Journal of Health and Social Behavior* 18 (March 1977): 54–61.

Conn, Robert H., and Anderson, Dudley. "D.C. Mounts Unfunded Program of Screening for Lead Poisoning." *HSMHA Health Report* 86 (May 1971): 409–13.

Croog, S., and Peters, N. "Health Beliefs and Smoking; Patterns in Heart Patients and Their Wives: A Longitudinal Study." *American Journal of Public Health* 67 (October 1977): 921–30.

Dalis, G. T., and Strasser, B. B. *Teaching Strategies for Values Awareness and Decision Making in Health Education.* Thorofare, N.J.: Slack, 1977.

Dallas, J. L. "Health Education: Enabler for a Higher Quality of Life." *Health Services Reports* 87, no. 10 (December 1972): 910–18.

Dalzell, Irene. "Evaluation of a Prenatal Teaching Program." *Nursing Research* 14 (Spring 1965): 160–63.

Danforth, N., and Swaboda, B. *Agency for International Development Health Education Study.* Washington, D.C.: Westinghouse Health Systems, March 17, 1978.

Deeds, S. G. *A Guidebook for Family Planning Education.* DHEW publication no. (HSA) 74-16002. Bureau of Community Health Services, 1973.

Delbecq, A. L.; Van de Ven, A. H.; and Gustafson, D. A. *Group Techniques for Program Planning.* Glenview, Ill.: Scott, Foresman, 1975.

Dershewitz, Robert A., and Williamson, John W. "Preventing of Childhood Household Injuries: A Controlled Clinical Trial." *American Journal of Public Health* 67 (December 1977): 1148–53.

Dominguez, A. V. "Stimulating Community Involvement Through Mass Organizations in Cuba: The Women's Role." *International Journal of Health Education* 20 (1977): 57–60.

D'Onofrio, C. N. "SOPHE and the Quality of Life." *Health Services Reports* 87, no. 10 (December 1972): 955–57.

Drummond, T. *Using The Method of Paulo Freire in Nutrition Education: An Experimental Plan for Community Action in Northeast Brazil.* Cornell International Nutrition Monograph Series, no. 3. Ithaca, N.Y.: Cornell University Press, 1975.

Eastman, C.; Randall, A.; and Hoffer, P. L. "How Much to Abate Pollution?" *Public Opinion Quarterly* 38 (Winter 1974–75): 574–84.

Edwards, Laura E., et al. "An Experimental Comprehensive High School Clinic." *American Journal of Public Health* 67 (August 1977): 765–66.

Elder, Carl A. *Making Value Judgements: Decisions of Today.* Chicago: Merrill, 1972.

Elwood, T. W.; Ericson, E.; and Lieberman, S. "Comparative Educational Approaches to Screening for Colorectal Cancer." *American Journal of Public Health* 68 (February 1978): 135–38.

Engel, J. F.; Wales, H. G.; and Warshaw, M. R. *Promotional Strategy.* Homewood, Ill; Irwin 1975.

Environmental Protection Agency. *The Quality of Life Concept: A Potential Tool for Decision-Makers.* March 1973.

Evans, R. I., et al. "Deterring the Onset of Smoking in Children: Knowledge of Immediate Physiological Effects and Coping with Peer Pressure, Media Pressure and Parent Modeling," *Journal of Applied Social Psychology* 8, no. 2 (1978): 126–35.

Faden, R. R., and Faden, A. I. *Ethical Issues in Public Health Policy: Health Education and Lifestyle Interventions. Health Education Monographs* 6, no. 2 (Summer 1978).

Farquhar, John W., et al. "Community Education for Cardiovascular Health." *Lancet* 1, no. 8023 (June 4, 1977): 1192–95.

Fass, M. F.; Green, L. W.; and Levine, D. M. "Design of an Experimental Intervention to Increase Family Reinforcement in the Home for Patient Compliance." Paper presented at the 103rd Annual Meeting of the American Public Health Association, November 1975, Chicago.

Fedder, D., and Beardsley, R. "Training Pharmacists to Become Patient Educators." Paper presented to the section of teachers of pharmacy administration of the annual meeting of the American Association of Colleges of Pharmacy, 18 July 1978, Orlando, Fla.

Feldman, M. E. "Learning by Programmed and Test Format at Three Levels of Difficulty." *Journal of Educational Psychology* 56 (1965): 133–39.

Figà-Talamanca, I. "Problems in the Evaluation of Training of Health Personnel." *Health Education Monographs* 3 (Fall 1975): 232–50.

Finkelstein, M. O.; Pickerel, P. A.; and Glasser, G. J. "The Death of Children: A

Nonparametric Statistical Analysis of Compensation for Anguish." *Columbia Law Review* 74 (June 1974): 884–93.

Fischer, D. W. "On the Problems of Measuring Environmental Benefits and Costs." *Social Science Information* 13 (April 1974): 95–105.

Fisher, A. A., et al. "Training Teachers in Population Education Institutes in Baltimore." *Journal of School Health* 46 (September 1976): 357–60.

Fisher, L. A., et al. "Collection of a Clean Voided Urine Specimen: A Comparison Among Spoken, Written, and Computer-based Instructions." *American Journal of Public Health* 67 (July 1977): 640–44.

Fletcher, J. E., and Thompson, H. B. "On the Problems of Measuring Environmental Benefits and Costs." *Social Science Information* 13 (April 1974): 95–105.

Flexner, W. A.; McLaughlin, C. P.; and Littlefield, J. E. "Discovering What the Health Consumer Really Wants." *Health Care Management Reviews* 2 (Fall 1977): 43–49.

Focal Points. Bureau of Health Education, DHEW, July 1977.

Focal Points. Bureau of Health Education, DHEW, September 1976.

Fonoroff, A., and Levin, L., eds. "Issues in Self-Care." *Health Education Monographs* 5 (Summer 1977): 108–89.

Foreyt, J. P., ed. *Behavioral Treatment of Obesity.* Oxford: Pergamon, 1977.

Forward Plan For Health FY 1977–81. DHEW pub. no. (OS) 76–50024. Public Health Service, August 1975.

Fourteen Communities Survey, February 1973–June 1974, Hypertension Detection and Follow-Up Study National Heart, Lung and Blood Institute. Quoted in *The National High Blood Pressure Month Book,* May 1977. NHBPEP, DHEW pub. no. (NIH) 77–1216. 1977.

Freedman, J. L.; Carlsmith, J. M.; and Sears, D. Q. *Social Psychology.* Englewood Cliffs, N.J.: Prentice-Hall, 1970.

Freeman, R. B. *Community Health Nursing Practice.* Philadelphia: Saunders, 1970.

French, W. L., and Bell, C. H., *Organizational Development: Behavioral Science Interventions for Organization Improvement.* Englewood Cliffs, N.J.: Prentice-Hall, 1973.

Friedman, M., and Rosenman, R. *Type A Behavior and Your Heart.* New York: Knopf, 1974.

Gaines, M. J. "An Evaluation of Three Methods of Teaching Freshmen Health Education." *Journal of the American College Health Association* 13 (February 1965): 347–55.

Gilmore, G. D. "Needs Assessment Processes for Community Health Education." *International Journal of Health Education* 20 (1977): 164–73.

Glaser, B. G., and Strauss, A. L. *Grounded Theory.* Chicago: Aldine, 1965.

Good, C. V., ed. *Foundations in Education: Dictionary of Education.* New York: McGraw-Hill, 1959.

Gordis, L.; Markowitz, M.; and Lilienfeld, A. "The Inaccuracy of Using Interviews to Estimate Patient Reliability in Taking Medications at Home." *Medical Care* 7 (1969): 49–54.

Grant, R. H. "Family and Self-Help Education in Isolated Rural Communities." *Health Education Monographs* 5 (Summer 1977): 143–60.

Green, L. W. "Should Health Education Abandon Attitude Change Strategies? Perspectives from Recent Research." *Health Education Monographs* 1, no. 30 (1970): 25–48.

Green, L. W. "Toward Cost-Benefit Evaluations of Health Education: Some Concepts, Methods and Examples." *Health Education Monographs* 2, supplement no. 1 (1974): 34–64.

Green, L. W. "Educational Strategies to Improve Compliance with Preventive and Therapeutic Regimens: The Recent Evidence." In *Compliance in Health Care,* edited by R. B. Haynes, D. Sackett, and W. Taylor. Baltimore: Johns Hopkins University Press, 1979.

Green, L. W. "Diffusion and Adoption of Innovations Related to Cardiovascular Risk Behavior in the Public." In *Applying Behavioral Science to Cardiovascular Risk,* edited by A. J. Enelow and J. B. Henderson. New York: American Heart Association, 1975.

Green, L. W. "Evaluation and Measurement: Some Dilemmas for Health Education." *American Journal of Public Health* 67 (February 1977): 155–61.

Green, L. W. "Determining the Impact and Effectiveness of Health Education As It Relates to Federal Policy." *Health Education Monographs* 6, supplement no. 1 (Spring 1978): 28–66.

Green, L. W. "Quality in Patient Education. What Is It and How Do We Measure It?" In *National Symposium on Patient Education, September 24–26, 1977, Proceedings.* Atlanta: Bureau of Health Education, Center for Disease Control, 1978.

Green, L. W., et al. *The Dacca Family Planning Experiment: A Comparative Evaluation of Programs Directed at Males and at Females,* Pacific Health Education Reports, no. 3. Berkeley: University of California Press, 1972.

Green, L. W., et al. "Research and Demonstration Issues in Self-care: Measuring the Decline of Medicocentrism." *Health Education Monographs* 5 (1977): 161–89.

Green, L. W., et al. *Guidelines for Health Education in Maternal and Child Health. International Journal of Health Education* 21 (supplement), no. 3 (July–September 1978): 1–33.

Green, L. W., et al. "Development of Randomized Patient Education Experiments with Urban Poor Hypertensives." *Patient Counseling and Health Education* (Excerpta Medica), 1 (Winter/Spring 1979): 106–11.

Green, L. W., and Faden, R. R. "Patient-Package Inserts: Potential Impact on Patients." *Drug Information Journal* 2 (January 1977): 64s–70s, (supplement).

Green, L. W., and Kansler, C. *The Scientific and Professional Literature on Patient Education.* Detroit: Gale Information Service, 1979.

Green, L. W., and Krotki, K. J. "Class and Parity Biases in Family Planning Programs: The Case of Karachi." *Eugenics Quarterly (Social Biology)* 15 (December 1968): 235–51.

Green, L. W.; Levine, D. M.; and Deeds, S. G. "Clinical Trials of Health Education for Hypertensive Outpatients: Design and Baseline Data." *Preventive Medicine* 4 (1975): 417–25.

Green, L. W.; Lewis F. M.; and Levine, D. M. "The Complementarity of Statistical Profiles, Clinical Judgement, and Behavioral Theory in the Diagnosis of Patient Educational Needs." Paper presented at the Second Annual Needs Assessment Conference, 28 March, 1978. Louisville, Ky.

Griffiths, W., and Knutson, A. L. "The Role of Mass Media in Public Health." *American Journal of Public Health* 50 (April 1960): 515–23.

Hamilton, V. E. "Community Resource Development: Health Education Programs in North Carolina." In *Proceedings: Extension Seminar on Health Education and Rural Health Care Research Forum* edited by B. L. Bible. Chicago: American Medical Association, 1976.

Havelock, R. G., and Havelock, M. G. *Training for Change Agents.* Ann Arbor: Institute for Social Research, University of Michigan Press, 1973.

Health Education Center. *Strategies for Health Education in Local Health Departments.* Baltimore: Maryland State Department of Health and Mental Hygiene, 1977.

Health Education Strategies for Hypertension Control." National Heart, Lung, and Blood Institute grant no. 1R25HL17016, co-principle investigators L. W. Green and D. M. Levine. Johns Hopkins Health Services Research and Development Center, 1974.

The Health and Nutrition Examination Survey 1971 (preliminary data). DHEW pub. no. (NIH) 77–1216. National High Blood Pressure Education Program, 1977.

Heit, P. "The Berkeley Model." *Health Education* 8 (January–February 1977): 2–3.

Henderson, V., and Nite, G. *Principles and Practice of Nursing.* New York: Macmillan, 1978.

Hochbaum, G. M. *Public Participation in Medical Screening Programs: A Socio-Psychological Study.* Public Health Service pub. no. 572. 1959.

Hypertension Detection and Follow-Up Program Cooperation Group. "Race, Education and Prevalence of Hypertension." *American Journal of Epidemiology* 106 (1971): 351–61.

Hypertension and Hypertensive Heart Disease in Adults, United States, 1960–62. National Health Survey, National Center for Health Statistics, series 11, no. 13, 1966.

Inter-Society Commission for Heart Disease Resources, Atherosclerosis Study Group and Epidemiology Study Group. "Primary Prevention of the Atherosclerotic Diseases." *Circulation* 42 (1970): A55.

Inter-Society Commission for Heart Disease Resources, Atherosclerosis Study Group and Epidemiology Study Group. "Guidelines for the Detection, Diagnosis, and Management of Hypertensive Populations." *Circulation* 44 (1971): A263, rev. August 1972.

Inui, T. S. "Effects of Post-Graduate Physician Education on the Management and Outcomes of Patients with Hypertension." Master of Science Thesis, Johns Hopkins University School of Hygiene and Public Health, 1973.

Jaffe, F. S. "Short-term Costs and Benefits of United States Family Planning Programs." *Studies in Family Planning* 5 (March 1974): 98–105.

James, G. "The Effects of a Health Activation Program on Junior High School Students in Utah." *Health Education Monographs* 5 (Winter 1977): 380–81 (abstract).

Jencks, S., and Green, L. W. "Developing a Hospital-based Patient Education Program." *Quality Review Bulletin* 4 (October 1978): 8–11.

Jenkins, C. D. "Components of the Coronary-prone Behavior Pattern—New Relations to Silent Myocardial Infarction and Blood Lipids." *Journal of Chronic Disease* 19 (1966): 599–609.

Jessor, R. "Predicting Time of Onset of Marijuana Use: A Developmental Study of High School Youth." In *Predicting Adolescent Drug Abuse: A Review of Issues, Methods and Correlates,* edited by D. J. Lettieri. National Institute of Drug Abuse, 1975.

Johnston, H. C. "Health Education in the Extension Service: A Historical Perspective." *Health Education Monographs* 3 (Spring 1975): 13–25.

Kanaaneh, H. A. K., et al. "The Eradication of a Large Scabies Outbreak Using Community-wide Health Education." *American Journal of Public Health* 66 (June 1976): 564–67.

Kandel, D. "Some Comments on the Relationship of Selected Criterion Variables to Adolescent Drug Use." In *Predicting Adolescent Drug Abuse: A Review of Issues, Methods and Correlates,* edited by D. J. Lettieri. National Institute of Drug Abuse, 1975.

Kaplan, R. "Teaching Problem-Solving with Television to College Freshmen in Health Education." Ph.D. thesis, Ohio State University, 1962.

Kaplun, A., and R. Erben, eds. *Health Education in Europe.* 2d ed. Geneva: *International Journal of Health Education,* 1976.

Katz, R. C., and Zlutnick, S., eds. *Behavior Therapy and Health Care Principles and Applications.* New York: Pergamon, 1975.

Kazdin, A. E. *Behavior Modification in Applied Settings.* Homewood, Ill.: Dorsey, 1975.

Kegeles, S. S. "Why People Seek Dental Care: A Test of a Conceptual Formulation." *Journal of Health and Human Behavior* 4 (Fall 1963): 166–73.

Kelman, H. "Attitudes Are Alive and Well and Gainfully Employed in the Sphere of Action." *American Psychologist* 29 (May 1974): 310–24.

Kirscht, J. P. "The Health Belief Model and Illness Behavior." *Health Education Monographs* 2 (1974): 387–408.

Knott, R. C. "Health Activities Project—A Different Approach." Paper presented at the annual meeting of the American School Health Association, October 1977, Atlanta.

Knowles, J. "The Responsibility of the Individual." *Daedalus* 106 (Winter 1977): 57–80.

Kohlberg, L. "Cognitive-Developmental Approach to Moral Education." *The Humanist* 32, no. 6 (November–December 1972): 13–16.

Kosa, J.; Antonovsky, A.; and Zola, I. K., eds. *Poverty and Health: A Sociological Analysis.* Cambridge, Mass.: Harvard University Press, 1969.

Kreuter, M. "An Interaction Model to Facilitate Awareness and Behavior Change." *Journal of School Health* 46 (November 1976): 543–45.

Kreuter, M. "Health Activation: Personal Responsibility in Prevention." In *Proceedings of the 12th Annual Prospective Medicine Conference.* San Diego: Society for Prospective Medicine, 1977.

Kreuter, M. W., and Green, L. W. "Evaluation of School Health Education: Identifying Purpose, Keeping Perspective." *Journal of School Health* 48 (April 1978): 228–35.

Kunstel, F. "Assessing Community Needs: Implications for Curriculum and Staff Development in Health Education." *Journal of School Health* 48 (April 1978): 220–24.

Kupst, M. J., et al. "Evaluation of Methods to Improve Communication in the Physician-Patient Relationship." *American Journal of Orthopsychiatry* 45 (April 1975): 420–29.

Kwon, E. Hyock "Use of the Agent System in Seoul." *Studies in Family Planning* 2 (November 1971): 327–40.

LaLonde, M. *A New Perspective on the Health of Canadians.* Ottawa, Canada. Ministry of National Health and Welfare, 1974.

Lanese, R. R., and Thrush, R. S. "Measuring Readability of Health Education Literature." *Journal of American Dietetic Association* 42 (March 1963): 214–17.

Lazes, P. M., et al. "Improving Patient Care Through Participation: The Newark Experiment in Staff and Patient Involvement." *International Journal of Health Education* 20 (1977): 61–68.

Leventhal, H., and Singer, R. P. "Affect Arousal and Positioning of Recommendations in Persuasive Communications." *Journal of Personality and Social Psychology* 4 (1966): 137–46.

Levin, L.; Katz, A.; and Holst, E. *Self Care: Lay Initiatives in Health.* New York: Prodist, 1976.

Levine, D. M., et al. "Health Education for Hypertensive Patients." *Journal of American Medical Association* 241 (April 20, 1979): 1700–03.

Lewin, K. "Studies in Group Decision." In *Group Dynamics, Research and Theory,* edited by D. Cartwright and A. Zander. Evanston, Ill.: Row, Peterson, 1953.

Lieberman, S. S. "The Isfahan Communication Project." *Studies in Family Planning* 4 (April 1973): 87–91.

Linsky, A. S. "Stimulating Responses to Mailed Questionnaires: A Review." *Public Opinion Quarterly* 39 (Spring 1975): 82–101.

Linstone, H. A., and Turoff, M. *The Delphi Method: Techniques and Applications.* Reading, Mass.: Addison-Wesley, 1975.

Long, Lillian D. "The Evaluation of Continuing Education Efforts." *American Journal of Public Health* 59 (June 1969): 967–73.

Lubin, B., and Eddy, W. B. "The Laboratory Training Model: Rationale, Method, and Some Thoughts for the Future." In *Sensitivity Training and the Laboratory Approach: Readings About Concepts and Applications,* edited by R. T. Colembiewski and A. Blumberg. Itasca, Ill., Peacock, 1973.

McAlister, A. L., et al. "Behavioral Science Applied to Cardiovascular Health: Progress and Research Needs in the Modification of Risk-taking Habits in Adult Populations." *Health Education Monographs* 4 (Spring 1976): 45–74.

McAlister, A. "Systematic Peer Leadership to Discourage Onset of Tobacco Dependency." Paper presented at the annual meeting of the American Psychological Association, August 1978, Toronto.

Maccoby, N., et al. "Reducing the Risk of Cardiovascular Disease: Effects of a Community-based Campaign on Knowledge and Behavior." *Journal of Community Health* 3 (Winter 1977): 100–114.

McGuire, W. J. "Communication-Persuasion Models for Drug Education." In *Research on Methods and Programs of Drug Education,* edited by Michael Goodstadt. Toronto: Addiction Research Foundation, 1978.

McTaggart, A. C. "The Readability of Health Textbooks." In *Synthesis of Research in Selected Areas of Health Instruction,* edited by C. H. Veenker. Washington, D.C.: National Education Association, 1963.

Mahoney, M. J. *Cognition and Behavior Modification.* Cambridge, Mass.: Ballinger, 1974.

Mahoney, M. J. *Cognitive Behavior Modification.* New York: Ballinger, 1977.

Maiman, L.; Green, L. W.; and Gibson, G. "Education for Self-Treatment by Adult Asthmatics." *Journal of the American Medical Association,* 241 (May 4, 1979): 1919–22.

Meadows, D. "Patients Learn About Diabetes from Teaching Machines." *Hospitals: JAHA* 39 (December, 1965): 77–82.

Mechanic, D. "The Influence of Mothers on Their Children's Health Attitudes and Behavior." *Pediatrics* 33 (March 1964): 44–53.

Medis, L. P., and Fernando, P. A. "Health Education in Emergency Situations: A Cholera Outbreak in Sri Lanka." *International Journal of Health Education* 20 (1977): 200–04.

Mendelsohn, H. "Mass Communications and Cancer Control." In *Cancer: The Behavioral Dimensions,* edited by J. W. Cullen, et al. New York: Raven, 1976.

Mersky, H. "Assessment of Pain." *Physiotherapy* 60 (April 1974): 96–98.

Metsch, J. M., et al. "The Impact of Training on Consumer Participation in the Delivery of Health Services." *Health Education Monographs* 3 (Fall 1975): 251–61.

Mico, P. R., and Ross, H. S. *Health Education and Behavioral Science.* Oakland: Third Party, 1975.

Milio, N. *The Care of Health in Communities: Access for Outcasts.* New York: Macmillan, 1975.

Milio, N. "A Framework for Prevention: Changing Health-Damaging to Health-Generating Life Patterns." *American Journal of Public Health,* (May 1976): 435–39.

Minkler, M. "The Use of Incentives in Family Planning Programmes." *International Journal of Health Education* 19, supplement no. 3 (1976).

Moriyama, I. M.; Krueger, D. E.; and Stamler, J. *Cardiovascular Diseases in the United States.* Cambridge, Mass.: Harvard University Press, 1971.

Mucchielli, R. *Introduction to Structural Psychology.* New York: Funk & Wagnalls, 1970.

Mueller, M. "HMO Act of 1973." Social Security Administration, Office of Research and Statistics, Note no. 5, 1974.

Mullen, P. D. "Cutting Back: An Overview." *Health Education Monographs,* in press.

National Center for Health Services. *Infant Mortality Rates: Socio-economic Factors,* U.S. DHEW, March 1972.

National Center for Health Statistics. *Blood Pressure of Persons 6–74 years of age in the United States.* NCHS Advance Data no. 1, October 18, 1976.

Navarro, V. *Medicine Under Capitalism.* New York: Prodist, 1976.

Needle, R., and Swawlewitz, K. "A Study of Work and the Workplace: Implications of the Psychosocial Aspects for Health Education and an Occupational Health and Safety Program on a University Campus." Paper presented at the annual meeting of the American College Health Association, 1978, New Orleans.

Neill, J. S., and Bond, J. O. *Hillsborough County Oral Polio Vaccine Program.* Florida State Board of Health monograph no. 6. Jacksonville: Florida State Board of Health, 1964.

Neufeld, V. R. "Patient Education: A Critique." In *Compliance with Therapeutic Regimens,* edited by D. L. Sackett and R. B. Haynes. Baltimore: Johns Hopkins University Press, 1976.

The Nursing Development Conference Group. *Concept Formalization in Nursing: Process and Product.* Boston: Little, Brown, 1973.

Oettinger, A. G. *Run, Computer, Run! The Mythology of Educational Innovation.* Cambridge: Harvard University Press, 1969.

Osgood, G. E.; Suci, G. J.; and Tannenbaum, P. H. *The Measurement of Meaning.* Urbana: University of Illinois Press, 1961.

Osman, J. "The Use of Selected Value Clarifying Strategies in Health Education." *Journal of School Health* 54 (January 1974): 21–25.

Owen, S. G., et al. "Programmed Learning in Medical Education." *Postgraduate Medical Journal* 41 (1965): 201.

Parcel, G. S. "Skills Approach to Health Education: A Framework for Integrating Cognitive and Affective Learning." *Journal of School Health* 66 (1976): 403–6.

Parker, Alberta. *The Team Approach to Primary Care.* Neighborhood Health Center Seminar Program Monograph Series no. 3. Berkeley: University of California, January 1972.

Partridge, Kay B. "Planning a Health Education Program. The Critical Role of Situational Analysis." *Proceedings. Patient Education Workshop,* Health Education Center, 29 October, 1975, pp. 9–22. Baltimore: Health Education Center, Maryland State Department of Health and Mental Hygiene, 1976.

Peters, Ruanne, et al. "Daily Relaxation Response Breaks in a Working Population: II. Effects on Blood Pressure." *American Journal of Public Health* 67 (October 1977): 954–59.

Phillips, James F., et al. "An Experiment with Payment, Quota, and Clinic Affiliation Schemes for Lay Motivators in the Philippines." *Studies in Family Planning* 6 (September 1975): 326–34.

Polgar, S. "Health Actions in Cross-Cultural Perspective." In *Handbook of Medical Sociology,* edited by H. E. Freeman, S. Levine, and L. G. Reeder. Englewood Cliffs, N.J.: Prentice-Hall, 1963.

Putting Knowledge to Use: A Distillation of the Literature Regarding Knowledge Transfer and Change. Los Angeles, Calif.: Human Interaction Research Institute, 1976.

Pyrczak F., and Roth D. H. "The Readability of Directions on Nonprescription Drugs." *Journal of American Pharmacology Association* 16 (1976): 242–43, 267.

Radke, M., and Caso, E. K. "Lecture and Discussion-Decision As Methods of Influencing Food Habits." *Journal of the American Dietetic Association.* 24 (January 1948): 23–31.

Redman, B. K. *The Process of Patient Teaching in Nursing.* 3d ed. St. Louis: Mosby, 1976.

Reeder, L. G.; Ramacher, L.; and Gorednik, S. *The Handbook on Scales and Indices.* Santa Monica, Calif.: Goodyear, 1976.

Reinhardt, A. M., and Chatlin, E. D. "Assessment of Health Needs in a Community: The Basis for Program Planning." In *Current Practices in Family-Centered Community Nursing,* edited by A. M. Reinhardt and M. D. Quinn. St. Louis: 1977, 138–90.

Reinhardt, A. M., and Quinn, M. D., eds. *Current Practices in Family-Centered Community Nursing.* Vol. 1. St. Louis: Mosby, 1977.

Reinhart, R., and Cazavelan, J. "Mental Health Consumer Survey on a Shoestring Budget—It Is Possible!" *American Journal of Community Psychology* 3 (September 1975): 273–76.

Report of the President's Committee on Health Education. New York: Public Affairs Institute, 1973.

Richards, D. N. "Methods and Effectiveness of Health Education: The Past, Present and Future of Social Scientific Involvement." *Social Science and Medicine* 9 (1975): 141–56.

Roberts, Beryl J., et al. "An Experimental Study of Two Approaches to Communication." *American Journal of Public Health* 53 (September 1963): 1361–81.

Robertson, H. R. "Removing Barriers to Health Care." *Nursing Outlook* 17 (September 1969): 43–46.

Robinson, Emerson. "A Comparative Evaluation of the Scrub and Brush Methods of Toothbrushing with Flossing As an Adjunct (in Fifth- and Sixth-Graders)." *American Journal of Public Health* 66 (November 1976): 1078–81.

Rogers, E. M. *Communication Strategies for Family Planning.* New York: Free Press, 1973.

Rogers, E. M., and Shoemaker, F. F. *Communication of Innovations: A Cross-Cultural Approach.* 2d ed. New York: The Free Press, 1972.

Rogers-Warren, A., and Warren, S. F. *Ecological Perspectives in Behavior Analysis.* Baltimore: University Park, 1977.

Rokeach, M. *Beliefs, Attitudes and Values: A Theory of Organization and Change.* San Francisco: Jossey-Bass, 1970.

Roos, Noralou P. "Evaluating Health Programs: Where Do We Find the Data?" *Journal of Community Health* 1 (Fall 1975): 39–51.

Rosenblatt, Daniel, and Kabasakalian, Levon. "Evaluation of Venereal Disease Information Campaign for Adolescents." *American Journal of Public Health* 56 (July 1966): 1104–14.

Rosenstock, I. M. "Why People Use Health Services." *Milbank Memorial Fund Quarterly* 44 (July 1966): 94–127.

Rosenstock, I. M. "Historical Origins of the Health Belief Model." *Health Education Monographs* 2 (1974): 328–35.

Rosenstock, I. M. "General Criteria for Evaluating Health Education Programs." In *Proceedings of the National Heart and Lung Institute Working Conference on Health Behavior.* DHEW pub. no. (NIH) 76-868. 1975.

Roter, D. L. "Patient Participation in the Patient-Provider Interaction: The Effects of Patient Question-Asking on the Quality of Interaction, Satisfaction and Compliance." *Health Education Monographs* 5 (Winter 1977): 281–315.

Rothman, J. "Three Models of Community Organization Practice." In *Strategies of Community Organization: A Book of Readings,* edited by F. M. Cox et al. Itasca, Ill.: Peacock, 1970.

Rothman, J.; Erlich, J. L.; and Teresa, J. G. *Promoting Innovation and Change in Organizations and Communities.* New York: Wiley, 1976.

Rubin, I.; Plovnick, M.; and Fry, R. "Initiating Planned Changes in Health Care Systems." *Journal of Applied Behavioral Science* 10 (1974): 107–24.

Russell, R. D. *Health Education.* Washington, D.C.: National Education Association, 1975.

Ruth, V., and Partridge, K. B. "Community Health Nursing: Differences in Perception of Education and Practice." *Nursing Outlook* 26 (October 1978): 622–28.

Rymer, S. "A Community Health Representative Program." *Health Education* 7 (November–December 1976): 17–19.

Sackett, D. L., and Haynes, R. B., eds. *Compliance with Therapeutic Regimens.* Baltimore: Johns Hopkins University Press, 1976.

Sayegh, J., and Green, L. W. "Family Planning Education: Program Design, Training Component and Cost-Effectiveness of a Postpartum Program in Beirut." *International Journal of Health Education* 19 (January–March 1976): 1–20 (supplement).

Schlotfeldt, R. "This I Believe . . . Nursing Is Health Care." *Nursing Outlook* 30 (April 1972): 245.

Schnocks, H. Foreword to *Health Education in Europe,* 2d ed., edited by A. Kaplun and R. Erben. Geneva: *International Journal of Health Education,* 1976.

School Health Curriculum Project. DHEW pub. no. (CDC) 78-8359. December 1977.

Schramm, W. "Learning from Instructional Television." *Review of Educational Research* 32 (1962): 156–67.

Schulz, E. D. "Television Brings Drama to Clinic Patients." *American Journal of Nursing* 62 (1962): 98–99.

Sehnert, K., and Eisenberg, H. *How to Be Your Own Doctor Sometimes.* New York: Grosset & Dunlap, 1975.

Selye, H. *The Stress of Life.* New York: McGraw-Hill, 1956.

Simon, S.; Howe, L.; and Kirschenbaum, H. *Values Clarification: A Handbook of Practical Strategies for Teachers and Students,* New York: Hart, 1972.

Skinner, B. F. "Teaching Machines." *Science* 128 (1958): 969–77.

Slack, W. V., et al. "Dietary Interviewing by Computer: An Experimental Approach to Counseling." *Journal of American Dietetic Association* 69 (1976): 514–17.

Sleet, D. A., and Stadsklev, R. "Annotated Bibliography of Simulations and Games in Health Education." *Health Education Monographs* 5, supplement no. 1 (1977): 4–90.

Sliepcevich, E. M. *School Health Education Study: A Summary Report.* Washington, D.C.: School Health Education Study, 1964.

Sliepcevich, E. M. "Impressions of an Overviewer." In *Proceedings: Preparation and Practice of Community, Patient and School Health Educators.* DHEW, Bureau of Health Manpower, 1978.

Smith, P. B., et al. "The Medical Impact of an Antepartum Program for Pregnant Adolescents: A Statistical Analysis." *American Journal of Public Health* 68 (February 1978): 169–72.

Sobel, D., and Hornbacher, F. *An Everyday Guide to Your Health.* New York: Grossman, 1973.

Social Security Disability Applicant Statistics, 1968. DHEW pub. no. (SSA) 73-1911. Social Security Administration, Office of Research and Statistics, June 1972.

Society for Public Health Education. *Training. Health Education Monographs* 3 (Fall 1975).

Sorochan, W., and Bender, S. *Teaching Elementary Health Science.* Menlo Park, Calif.: Addison-Wesley, 1975.

Source Book of Health Insurance Data. Washington, D.C.: Health Insurance Institute, 1978.

Spiegel, Charlotte, V., and Lindaman, Francis C. "Children Can't Fly: A Program to Prevent Childhood Morbidity and Mortality from Window Falls." *American Journal of Public Health* 67 (December 1977): 143–47.

Stahl, Sidney, et al. "Motivational Interventions in Community Hypertension Screening." *American Journal of Public Health* 67 (April 1977): 345–52.

Stamler, J., et al. "Hypertension. The Problem and the Challenge." In *The Hypertension Handbook* West Point, Pa.: Merck Sharp & Dohme, 1971, pp. 3–29.

Steinberg, Sheldon S., and Fitzpatrick, Eugene D. "The Paducah Health Education Survey 1958." *American Journal of Public Health* 51 (May 1961): 732–45.

Stephens, J. M. *The Process of Schooling: A Psychological Examination.* New York: Holt, 1967.

Steuart, Guy W. "Planning and Evaluation in Health Education." *International Journal of Health Education* 12 (1969): 65–76.

Surgeon General's Scientific Advisory Committee on Television and Social Behavior. *Television and Growing Up: The Impact of Televised Violence.* Public Health Service, 1972.

Teenage Smoking: National Patterns of Cigarette Smoking, Ages 12 Through 17, in 1972 and 1974. DHEW pub. no. (NIH) 76-931. 1976.

Thoreson, C. E., and Mahoney, M. J. *Self-Control: Power to the Person.* Monterey, Calif.: Brooks/Cole, 1974.

Thorne, M. C., ed. *Consultation. Health Education Monographs* 4 (Winter 1975).

Tinkham, C. W., and Voorhies, E. F. *Community Health Nursing Evolution and Process.* New York: Appleton-Century-Crofts, 1972.

Tomic, B., et al. "Ivanjica: A Community Conquers Health." *International Journal of Health Education* 20 (April–June 1977): 1–16 (supplement).

Ubell, E. "Health Behavior Change: A Political Model." *Preventive Medicine* 1 (1972): 209–21.

Van Cura, L. J., et al. "Venereal Disease: Interviewing and Teaching by Computer." *American Journal of Public Health* 65 (1975): 1159–64.

Van de Ven, A. H., and Delbecq, A. L. "The Nominal Group As a Research Instrument for Exploratory Health Studies." *American Journal of Public Health* 62 (March 1972): 337–42.

Veenker, C. H., ed. *Synthesis of Research in Selected Areas of Health Instruction.* Washington, D.C.: National Education Association, 1963.

Veterans Administration Cooperative Study Group on Antihypertensive Agents: Effects of treatment on morbidity in hypertension.
   I. "Results in Patients with Diastolic Blood Pressures Averaging 115 Through 129 mm Hg." *Journal of American Medical Association* 202 (1967): 1028.

Veterans Administration Cooperative Study Group on Antihypertensive Agents: Effects of Treatment on Morbidity in Hypertension.
   II. "Results in Patients with Diastolic Blood Pressure Averaging 90 Through 114 mm Hg." *Journal of American Medical Association* 213 (1970): 1143.

Veterans Administration Cooperative Study Group on Antihypertensive Agents: Effects of Treatment on Morbidity in Hypertension.
   III. "Influence of Age, Diastolic Pressure, and Prior Cardiovascular Disease: Further Analysis of Side Effects." *Circulation* 45 (1972): 991.

Von Haden, H. I., and King, J. M. *Educational Innovators' Guide.* Worthington, Ohio: James, 1974.

Wallston, B. S., et al. "Development and Validation of the Health Locus of Control (HLC) Scale." *Journal of Consulting and Clinical Psychology* (August 1976): 580–85.

Wallston, K. A., and Wallston, B. S., eds. *Locus of Control and Health: A Review of the Literature.* Health Education Monographs 6, no. 2 (Spring 1978): 107–17.

Wang, V. L. "Application of Social Science Theories to Family Planning: Health Education in the People's Republic of China." *American Journal of Public Health* 66 (May 1976): 440–45.

Wang, V. L. "Social Goals, Health Policy and the Dynamics of Development As Bases for Health Education." *International Journal of Health Education* 20 (1977): 13–18.

Wang, V. L.; Ephross, P.; and Green, L.W. "The Point of Diminishing Returns in Nutrition Education Through Home Visits by Aides: An Evaluation of EFNEP." *Health Education Monographs* 3 (Spring 1975): 70–88.

Ward, G. H. "Changing Trends in Control of Hypertension." *Public Health Reports* 93 (January–February 1978): 31–34.

Warheit, G. J.; Bell, R. A.; and Schwab, J. J. *Needs Assessment Approaches: Concepts and Methods.* DHEW pub. no. (ADM) 77–472. National Institute of Mental Health, 1977.

Warner, Kenneth E. "The Effects of the Anti-Smoking Campaign on Cigarette Consumption." *American Journal of Public Health* 67 (July 1977): 645–50.

Watson, D. L., and Tharp, R. G. *Self-Directed Behavior—Self Modification for Personal Adjustment.* Monterey, Calif.: Brooks/Cole, 1977.

Wilkinson, G. S., et al. "Measuring Response to a Cancer Information Telephone Facility: Can-Dial." *American Journal of Public Health* 66 (April 1976): 367–71.

Williams, C. "Community Health Nursing—What Is It? *Nursing Outlook* 25 (April 1977): 250–54.

Williamson, John, et al. "Health Accounting: An Outcome-based System of Quality Assurance—Illustrative Applications to Hypertension." *Bulletin of the New York Academy of Medicine* 51 (1975): 727–38.

Wise, Harold, et al. *Making Health Teams Work.* Cambridge, Mass.: Ballinger, 1974.

Young, M. A. C. "Review of Research and Studies Related to Health Education (1961–1966): Communication Methods and Materials." *Health Education Monographs* 25 (1968): 1–70.

Young, M. A. C. "Review of Research and Studies Related to Health Education (1961–1966): Patient Education." *Health Education Monographs* 26 (1968): 1–64.

Young, M. A. C. "Review of Research and Studies Related to Health Education Practice (1961–1966): School Health Education." *Health Education Monographs* 28 (1969): 1–97.

Yura, H., and Walsh, M. B. *The Nursing Process.* 2d. ed. New York: Appleton-Century-Crofts, 1973.

Zaltman, Gerald, and Duncan, Robert. *Strategies for Planned Change.* New York: Wiley, 1977.

Zimmerman, B. J., and Rosenthal, T. L. "Observational Learning of 'Rules' Governed Behavior by Children." *Psychological Bulletin* 81 (1974): 29–42.

Index

56–64; behavioral targets for,
62–64; and changeability of
behaviors, 59–62; dimensions of, as
health problem, 41–46; inventory of
behaviors related to, 57–58; and
male mortality rates, 191–92, 193;
nonbehavioral causes of, 56–57;
rating importance of behaviors in,
58–59, 60 table. *See also*
Hypertension
Cartwright, D., 71–72
Caso, E.K., 101
Cauffman, J.E., 96
Certification, 134
Changeability of behavior, 59–62,
81–82; attribute method of
assessing, 60–62; high, 60, 62 table;
low, 60, 62 table
Chatlin, E.D., 163
Child-abuse prevention program:
objectives of, 229–31; predisposing,
enabling, and reinforcing factors for
physicians in, 226–29, 230; rationale
for, 225–26
Children, low-income: dental health
education for, 237–46
Cholesterol intake, control of, 56, 57,
61 table, 135
Classical conditioning, 101–2
Climate, 54
Coal miners, 55
Community development: as
educational strategy, 88, 103–4,
114; administrative considerations
in, 111–12 table; in community
demonstration project, 180–81; and
determinants of health, 109–10
table; and enabling factors, 88–89;
and health behavior, 108 table; and
health problems, 107 table; and
predisposing factors, 89; and
reinforcing factors, 89
Community health nursing, 163–65
Computer-aided instruction, 96, 97
Consultation, 105
Cornell Psychiatric Index, 233
Counseling. *See* Health counseling;
Individual instruction

Croog, S., 70
Crowder, Norman, 97
Curriculum development: PRECEDE
framework for, 145–46; in school
health education, 144–45

Delbecq, A.L., 24, 25
Delphi method, 26–28
Dental health education program, 147
table, 148, 149 table, 150 table,
237–46; administrative diagnosis of,
245–46; educational diagnosis of,
239–43; educational strategies in,
243–45; enabling factors in, 240–41
table; funding problems in, 246;
objectives of, 239, 240–41 table,
242 table; predisposing factors in,
240–41 table; reinforcing factors in,
240–41 table; restricted objectives
of, 48
Diabetes, 48, 56, 57
Diet: counseling about, 8; and
modeling, 101; and prenatal care,
233, 236, 238 table
Diffusion process, 81–84; and
educational strategies, 110 table;
learning objectives keyed to, 82–84;
role of mass media in, 92; theory
of, 81–82
Direct mail, 92, 93, 95 table
Disability, 41
Door-to-door requests, 94
Drug abuse, 148, 149 table, 150 table;
programs for, 30; reinforcing
factors in, 76

Educational diagnosis, 13, 14 fig.,
16–17, 68–85; and "blaming the
victim," 77; in community
demonstration project, 176–80,
182–84, 185; in dental health
education program, 239–43; and
diffusion of innovations, 81–84; and
educational strategies, 106, 108–10
tables; of hypertension, 198–206;
and learning objectives, 82–84; and
multicausal model, 69–70, 71 fig.,
76; in occupational health program,

prevention, 225–26, 227, 228 table; and hypertension control, 195, 196, 200, 203

Regulatory agencies, 213–14

Reinforcing factors, 13, 14 fig., 16, 76; in child-abuse prevention programs, 228 table, 229; in community demonstration project, 178–79; defined, 69, 70, 71 fig.; in dental health education program, 240–41 table; and educational strategies, 89, 106, 109–10 table, 114; and hypertension, 196–97, 198 fig., 199, 201–2, 203, 205, 206, 207; identifying and sorting, 77–78, 79 table; mass media as, 81–82; in maternal health education program, 232, 233, 237, 238 table; in occupational health program, 221, 223 table, 224 table; in school health education program, 155–57; setting priorities for, 78–81; and streptococcal throat infections, 79 table

Reinhardt, A.M., 163

Residence, 54

Resources: allocation of, 118–21; improved use of, 19–20

Responsive Education, 237, 239, 245

Richards, D.N., 5

Rokeach, M., 81

Role playing. *See* Simulations

Rosenstock, I.M., 6, 72–73

Ross, H.S., 105

Roter, D.L., 100

Schedule of Recent Experience, 233

Schlotfeldt, R., 160

Schnocks, H., 4

School Health Curriculum Project, 144–45, 154

School Health education programs, 142–58; accountability in, 151, 155–57; behavioral diagnosis in, 150–51; change in behavior as problematic goal of, 150–52, 153, 155; curriculum development of, 144–45; and "disease" orientation,

156; educational strategies for, 113; epidemiological diagnosis in, 146–50; evaluation of, 135, 151–53, 154, 155–57; individual instruction in, 90; knowledge and skills as goal of, 154–57; knowledge as predisposing factor in, 72; PRECEDE framework for, 145–46, 155–57; reinforcement in, 76; resources inadequate in, 152–53; social diagnosis in, 146–50

School Health Education Study, 144

Schramm, W., 98

Sedentary life-style, 56, 57

Self-care, 30–31, 104

Semantic differential, 74–75

Simulations: as educational strategy, 88, 99; administrative considerations in, 111–12 table; in dental health education, 245; and determinants of health, 109–10 table; and enabling factors, 89; and health behavior, 108 table; and health problems, 107 table; and predisposing factors, 89

Skills: in dental health education program, 237, 242–43 table; development of, 88, 89, 98–99; as enabling factors, 68, 71 fig., 75; as goal of school health education, 154–57; as learning objective, 82, 83 table; and predisposing factors, 89

Skinner, B.F., 97

Skydiving, 73, 74–75

Sleet, D.A., 99

Sliepcevich, E.M., 5

Small-group discussion: as educational strategy, 88, 100–101, 113, 114; administrative considerations in, 111–12 table; in dental health education, 243–45; and determinants of health, 109–10 table; effectiveness of, 98; and enabling factors, 89; and health behavior, 108 table; and health problems, 107 table; in hypertension control program, 206, 207–8, 209 table; to impart information, 89, 90; and